100 CASES IN

CLINICAL MEDICINE

JOHN REES MD FRCP
Consultant Physician and Senior Lecturer in Medicine,
Guy's, King's and St. Thomas' School of Medicine, London, UK

JAMES M. PATTISON MA DM MRCP
Consultant Nephrologist, Guy's and St. Thomas' Hospital, London, UK

GWYN WILLIAMS MD FRCP
Professor of Medicine, King's and St.Thomas' School of Medicine, London, UK

Hodder Arnold

A MEMBER OF THE HODDER HEADLINE GROUP

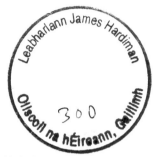

First published in Great Britain in 2000 by Arnold,
a member of the Hodder Headline Group
338 Euston Road, London NW1 3BH

http://www.hoddereducation.com

Distributed in the United States of America by
Oxford University Press Inc.
198 Madison Avenue, New York, NY10016
Oxford is a registered trademark of Oxford University Press

British Library Cataloguing in Publication Data
A catalogue record for this book is available from the British Library

Library of Congress Cataloging-in-Publication Data
A catalog record for this book is available from the Library of Congress

ISBN-10: 0 340 67702 3
ISBN-13: 978 0 340 67702 5

7 8 9 10

Commissioning Editor: Fiona Goodgame
Production Editor: James Rabson
Production Controller: Priya Gohil
Cover designer: Terry Griffiths

Typeset in 9/12 Helvetica by Saxon Graphics Ltd, Derby
Printed and bound in Great Britain by CPI, Bath

CONTENTS

PREFACE

Most doctors think that the most memorable way to learn medicine is to see patients. It is easier to recall information based on a real person than a page in a textbook. Another important element in the retention of information is the depth of learning. Learning that seeks to understand problems is more likely to be accessible later than superficial factual accumulation. This is the basis of problem based learning, where students explore problems with the help of a facilitator. The cases in this book are designed to provide another useful approach, parallel to seeing patients and giving an opportunity for self directed exploration of clinical problems. They are based on the findings of history taking and examination, together with the need to evaluate initial investigations such as blood investigations, X-rays and ECGs.

These cases are no substitute for clinical experience with real patients, but they provide a safe environment for students to explore clinical problems and their own approach to diagnosis and management. Most are common problems that might present to a general practitioner's surgery, a medical outpatients or a session on call in hospital. There are a few more unusual cases to illustrate specific points and to emphasize that rare things do present, even if they are uncommon. The cases are written to try to interest students in clinical problems and to enthuse them to find out more. They try to explore thinking about diagnosis and management of real clinical situations.

The cases cover a range of general medical problems. They are not in any particular order, to mimic the way patients present to surgery or Accident and Emergency departments. They can be dipped into or read through; they can be used by individuals or by groups as the starting point for self directed learning exercises. We hope they will be helpful but also stimulating and enjoyable, as all medicine should be.

John Rees
James M. Pattison
Gwyn Williams
January 2000

ACKNOWLEDGEMENTS

The authors would like to thank the following people for their help with illustrations:
Dr A. Saunders, Dr S. Rankin, Dr J. Reidy, Dr J. Bingham, Dr L. Macdonald,
Dr G. Cook, Dr T. Gibson, Professor R. Reznak.

A 72-year-old lady goes to her GP complaining of fatigue. Her husband has noticed that she has become increasingly lethargic and that she sleeps during the afternoon. This is out of character for her as she has always been very energetic. She also noticed that her bowel habit has changed and that she now tends to be constipated. Her hairdresser has commented that her hair seems to be thinning. Her mother had non-insulin-dependent diabetes mellitus.

On examination she has a slightly puffy facial appearance. Her skin is dry and scaling and her scalp hair is thinning. Her pulse is 52, regular, and blood pressure is 138/90. Examination of her heart, respiratory and abdominal systems is normal. Her neurological examination is unremarkable apart from tendon reflexes which react normally but relax slowly.

INVESTIGATIONS

		Normal
Haemoglobin	9.2 g/dl	(11.7–15.7 g/dl)
Mean cell volume	105 fl	(80–99 fl)
White cell count	4.2×10^9/l	($3.5–11.0 \times 10^9$/l)
Platelets	154×10^9/l	($150–440 \times 10^9$/l)
Sodium	142 mmol/l	(135–145 mmol/l)
Potassium	4.4 mmol/l	(3.5–5.0 mmol/l)
Urea	5.2 mmol/l	(2.5–6.7 mmol/l)
Creatinine	106 μmol/l	(70–120 μmol/l)
Glucose	4.9 mmol/l	(4.0–6.0 mmol/l)
Albumin	42 g/l	(35–50 g/l)
Urinalysis	NAD	

QUESTIONS

- What is the diagnosis?
- How would you investigate and manage this patient?

ANSWER 1

Chronic fatigue is a very common symptom with many causes. The differential diagnosis of chronic fatigue includes organ failure such as renal or cardiac failure, metabolic and endocrine abnormalities, underlying chronic infection or malignancy and depression. This patient has typical symptoms and signs of **hypothyroidism**. Hypothyroidism tends to present very insidiously. The symptoms may be present for many years before a diagnosis is made. She is lethargic and suffers from constipation, alopecia and anaemia. The skin is characteristically dry and scaly, and her scalp hair is sparse and brittle. Her pulse rate is slow. The apex beat may be difficult to locate due to the presence of a pericardial effusion. Slow relaxation of the ankle jerks is characteristic in severe cases. Hypothyroidism may have a psychiatric presentation – 'myxoedema madness'. The anaemia of hypothyroidism is usually a normochromic, normocytic anaemia, but may be macrocytic (as in this case) due to associated vitamin B_{12} deficiency. The most extreme presentation of hypothyroidism is myxoedema coma with severe bradycardia and hypothermia.

Her thyroid function tests are as follows: thyroid-stimulating hormone (TSH) 54 mU/l (<6 mU/l); free T4 2 pmol/l (9–22 pmol/l). The low free thyroxine level in this patient confirms hypothyroidism, and the elevated TSH implies primary thyroid pathology rather than hypopituitarism.

The commonest cause of primary hypothyroidism is autoimmune destruction of the thyroid gland. There may be a goitre palpable in Hashimoto's thyroiditis, or in a more chronic process the gland will be atrophied. In these causes thyroid autoantibodies are present.

! CAUSES OF HYPOTHYROIDISM

- Autoimmune destruction of the thyroid gland
- Post-thyroidectomy
- Post-^{131}I treatment for thyrotoxicosis
- Drugs for treatment of hypothyroidism – propylthiouracil, carbimazole
- Dietary iodine deficiency
- Inherited enzyme defects

This patient should have thyroid autoantibodies measured. In view of the macrocytic anaemia, vitamin B_{12} and gastric parietal antibodies should also be assayed. Replacement of the deficient thyroid hormones is the basis of treatment. Replacement is given in the form of thyroxine at a maintenance dose of 100–200 μg/day. The response is measured clinically and biochemically. Thyroid replacement therapy may precipitate cardiac ischaemia. In elderly patients and in those with cardiac disease, thyroxine replacement should be started cautiously at 25–50 μg/day and increased by 25–50 μg/day every three weeks.

A 28-year-old man complains of shortness of breath, cough and chest pain. The chest pain came on suddenly 6 hours previously when he was walking to work. It was a sharp pain in the left side of the chest. The pain was made worse by breathing. It settled over the next few hours and has left a mild ache in the left side on deep breathing. He felt a little short of breath at rest for the first hour or two after the pain came on but now only feels this on stairs or walking quickly. He has had a dry cough throughout the 6 hours.

He smokes 20 cigarettes a day and drinks 20 units of alcohol a week. He is on no medication. There is a previous history of a possible similar episode four years ago; he thinks that the pain was on the right side of the chest on that occasion. There is no relevant family history.

On examination he is a tall, thin man, not distressed or cyanosed. His pulse is 84/min and his blood pressure 128/78. His respiratory rate is 18/min. Heart sounds are normal. In the respiratory system the trachea and apex beat are not displaced. Expansion seems normal, as is percussion. There is decreased tactile vocal fremitus and softer breath sounds over the left side of the chest.

The chest X-ray is shown (Fig. 2.1).

QUESTIONS

- What does the X-ray show?
- What should be done now?

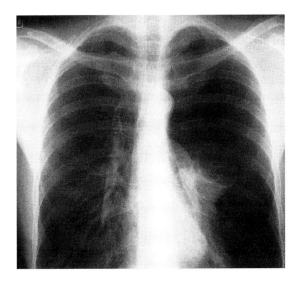

Figure 2.1 Chest X-ray

ANSWER 2

The chest X-ray shows a left **pneumothorax**. Pneumothoraces are usually visible on normal inspiratory films but an expiratory film may help when there is doubt. There is no mediastinal displacement on examination or X-ray to suggest a tension pneumothorax. Although he had symptoms initially, these have settled down as might be expected in a fit patient with no underlying lung disease and a small pneumothorax.

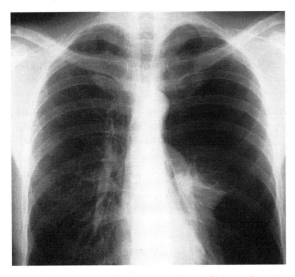

Figure 2.1 Chest X-ray showing mild-moderate left pneumothorax

The differential diagnosis of chest pain in a young man includes pneumonia and pleurisy, pulmonary embolism and musculoskeletal problems. However, the clinical signs and X-ray leave no doubt about the diagnosis in this man. Pneumothoraces are more common in tall, thin men, in smokers and in those with underlying lung disease. Further investigations such as computed tomography (CT) scan are not indicated unless there is a suggestion of underlying lung disease.

There is a suggestion that he may have had a similar episode in the past but it may have been on the right side. There is a tendency for recurrence of pneumothoraces, about 20 per cent after one event and 50 per cent after two. Because of this, pleurodesis should be considered after two pneumothoraces on the same side. In this man the first event is not documented and may have been on the other side so such intervention is not indicated.

The immediate management is to aspirate the pneumothorax through the second intercostal space anteriorly using a cannula of 16 Fr gauge or more, at least 3 cm long. Small pneumothoraces with no symptoms and no underlying lung disease can be left to absorb spontaneously but this is quite a slow process. Up to 2500 ml can be aspirated, stopping if it becomes difficult to aspirate or the patient coughs excessively. If the aspiration is unsuccessful or the pneumothorax recurs immediately, intercostal drainage to an underwater seal or valve may be indicated. Difficulties at this stage may require thoracic surgical intervention. This is considered earlier than it used to be since the adoption of less invasive video-assisted techniques.

KEY POINTS

- The patient should not be allowed to fly until the pneumothorax has resolved.
- The risk of recurrence will be reduced by stopping smoking.

CASE 3

A 75-year-old man is brought to hospital with an episode of dizziness. He still feels unwell at the time he is seen 30 min. after the onset. He has been well until the last six months. Over that time he has had some falls. These have occurred irregularly. On some occasions he has lost consciousness and he is unsure how long he has been unconscious. He has fallen and grazed his knees on a few occasions. On other occasions he has felt faint or dizzy and has had to sit down but has not lost consciousness. These episodes have usually happened on exertion but once or twice they have occurred while he is sitting down. He recovers over 10–15 min. after each episode. There is no history of chest pain or palpitations.

He lives alone and most of the episodes have not been witnessed. On one occasion his 20-year-old granddaughter was with him when he blacked out. She was very worried about him and called an ambulance. He looked so pale and still that she thought that he had died. He was taken to hospital but by this time he had recovered completely and was discharged home having been told that he had a normal ECG and chest X-ray.

In his previous medical history, he has had gout and some urinary frequency. A diagnosis of benign prostatic hypertrophy has been made and he is on no treatment for this. He takes ibuprofen occasionally when his gout gives him trouble. He used to smoke but stopped five years ago and he drinks 5–10 units of alcohol each week. The dizziness and blackouts have not been associated with alcohol consumption.

There is no relevant family history. He used to work as an electrician.

On examination, he is pale with a blood pressure of 96/64. The pulse rate is 33/min., regular. There are no murmurs on auscultation of the heart. The jugular venous pressure is raised 3 cm with occasional rises. There is no leg oedema; the peripheral pulses are palpable except for the left dorsalis pedis. The respiratory system is normal.

His ECG is shown (Fig. 3.1).

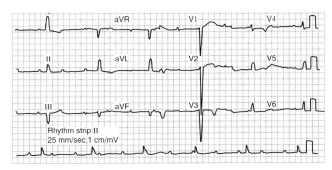

Figure 3.1

QUESTIONS

- What is the cause of his blackout?
- What does the ECG show?

ANSWER 3

The blackouts do not seem to have had any relationship to posture. They have been a mixture of dizziness and loss of consciousness. The one witnessed episode seems to have been associated with loss of colour. This suggests a loss of cardiac output usually associated with an arrhythmia. This may be the case despite the absence of any other cardiac symptoms. There may be an obvious flushing of the skin as cardiac output and blood flow return.

The normal ECG and chest X-ray when he attended hospital after an episode do not rule out an intermittent conduction problem. On this occasion the symptoms have remained in a more minor form. The ECG shows third degree or **complete heart block**. There is complete dissociation of the atrial rate and the ventricular rate which is 33/min. The episodes of loss of consciousness are called Stokes–Adams attacks and are caused by self-limited rapid tachyarrhythmias at the onset of heart block or transient asystole. Although these have been intermittent in the past he is now in stable complete heart block and, if this continues, the slow ventricular rate will be associated with reduced cardiac output which may cause fatigue, dizziness on exertion or heart failure. Intermittent failure of the escape rhythm may cause syncope.

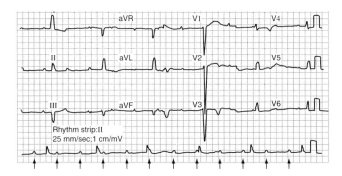

Figure 3.1 ECG showing complete heart block, p-waves arrowed.

On examination, the occasional rises in the jugular venous pressure are intermittent 'cannon' a-waves as the right atrium contracts against a closed tricuspid valve. In addition, the intensity of the first heart sound will vary.

The differential diagnosis of transient loss of consciousness splits into neurological and vascular causes. A witness is very helpful in differentiation. Neurological causes are various forms of epilepsy, often with associated features. Vascular causes are related to local or general reduction in cerebral blood flow. Local reduction may occur in transient ischaemic effects or vertebrobasilar insufficiency. A more global reduction, often with pallor, occurs with arrhythmias, postural hypotension and vasovagal faints.

The treatment should be insertion of a pacemaker. If the rhythm in complete heart block is stable then a permanent pacemaker should be inserted as soon as this can be arranged. This should be a dual-chamber system pacing atria then ventricles (DDD, dual sensing and pacing, triggered by atrial sensing, inhibited by ventricular sensing) or possibly a ventricular pacing system (VVI, pacing ventricle, inhibited by ventricular sensing). If there is doubt about the ventricular escape rhythm then a temporary pacemaker should be inserted immediately.

🔑 KEY POINTS

- When a patient suffers transient loss of consciousness, a careful history from a witness may help with the diagnosis.
- Normal examination and ECG do not rule out intermittent serious arrhythmias.
- Large waves in the jugular venous pressure are usually regular giant v-waves in tricuspid regurgitation or intermittent cannon a-waves in complete heart block.

CASE 4

A 58-year-old man presents to his GP complaining of a two-week history of progressive swelling of his legs. He feels otherwise well and has had no significant previous medical illnesses. He smokes 20 cigarettes per day and drinks 15 units of alcohol per week. He is taking no regular medication. On examination, there is marked pitting oedema of both legs extending up to the groin. His pulse is 72/min, regular, and blood pressure 140/90. His jugular venous pressure is not raised and heart sounds are normal with no added sounds. Examination of his respiratory, abdominal and neurological symptoms is normal.

INVESTIGATIONS

		Normal
Haemoglobin	14.6 g/dl	(13.3–17.7g/dl)
Mean cell volume	85 fl	(80–99 fl)
White cell count	7.2 × 10⁹/l	(3.9–10.6 × 10⁹/l)
Platelets	413 × 10⁹/l	(150–440 × 10⁹/l)
Sodium	138 mmol/l	(135–145 mmol/l)
Potassium	3.8 mmol/l	(3.5–5.0 mmol/l)
Urea	5.2 mmol/l	(2.5–6.7 mmol/l)
Creatinine	86 µmol/l	(70–120 µmol/l)
Albumin	18 g/l	(35–50g/l)
Glucose	4.5 mmol/l	(4.0–6.0 mmol/l)
Bilirubin	13 mmol/l	(3–17 mmol/l)
Alanine transaminase	33 iu/l	(5–35 iu/l)
Alkaline phosphatase	72 iu/l	(30–300 iu/l)
Cholesterol	13.2 mmol/l	(3.9–7.8 mmol/l)
Urinalysis	+++ protein; no blood	
24-hour urinary protein	12.6 g	(<200 mg/24 h)

QUESTIONS

- What do these findings indicate?
- What should be the management?

ANSWER 4

This patient presents with massive oedema but without any features of heart failure. The oedema with a low serum albumin and heavy proteinuria are diagnostic of the **nephrotic syndrome**. A working definition of the nephrotic syndrome is the presence of detectable oedema, proteinuria > 3.0 g/24 h and a serum albumin < 30 g/l. Severe oedema can also occur because of increased hydrostatic pressure in severe heart failure or venous obstruction, or because of hypoalbuminaemia in chronic liver disease or severe malnutrition.

Nephrotic syndrome is due to an increased leak of glomerular proteins, and may occur in primary glomerular disease or glomerular disease secondary to systemic disease.

❗ COMMON CAUSES OF NEPHROTIC SYNDROME IN ADULTS

Primary glomerular diseases	e.g. Membranous glomerulonephritis
	Minimal change disease
	Focal and segmental glomerulosclerosis
Systemic diseases	e.g. Diabetes mellitus
	Systemic lupus erythematosus (SLE)
	Amyloidosis

This patient should be referred to a nephrologist for further investigation and treatment. A renal biopsy is necessary to reach a histological diagnosis which is important as specific treatments for some of the above conditions are indicated. In this patient the biopsy showed membranous glomerulonephritis. This condition is usually idiopathic, but can be associated with carcinoma (bronchial/bowel especially), SLE, hepatitis B virus infection and certain drugs (e.g. gold, penicillamine). The patient should have a chest X-ray, faecal occult bloods, anti-DNA antibodies, complement levels and hepatitis B serology performed. The treatment for idiopathic membranous glomerulonephritis is controversial as it can remit and relapse spontaneously. Intensive immunosuppression is reserved for patients with a very low serum albumin (as in this case) or with rapidly deteriorating renal function. Patients with a serum albumin < 20 g/l are usually anticoagulated with warfarin as they are particularly susceptible to thromboembolism.

The major complications of nephrotic syndrome are infection, hypercholesterolaemia (as in this case), arterial and venous thromboses, acute renal failure (due either to overvigorous diuresis or rarely as a complication of minimal change disease) and chronic renal failure due to progression of the underlying glomerular disease.

⚷ KEY POINTS

- Leg oedema is related to increased hydrostatic pressure, reduced oncotic pressure or local obstruction to drainage.
- In adults with nephrotic syndrome, a renal biopsy is indicated.

CASE 5

An 82-year-old man has been in a residential home for three years since his wife died. He was unable to look after himself at home because of some osteoarthritis in the hips limiting his mobility. Apart from his reduced mobility, which has restricted him to a few steps on a frame and a rather irritable temper, he has had no problems in the residential care.

He has been referred to the visiting doctor because he has become much more difficult over 36 hours. He has accused the staff of assaulting him and stealing his money. He has been trying to get out of his bed and his chair, and this has resulted in a number of falls. On some occasions his speech has been difficult to understand. He has been incontinent of urine three times in the last 24 hours. Prior to this he has been incontinent on one or two occasions in the last six months.

When seen by the doctor he is rather sleepy but when roused seems frightened and verbally aggressive. He thinks that his money has been stolen by the staff and by policemen he has seen in his room. He is disorientated in place and time although reluctant to try to answer these questions.

He is a non-smoker and non-drinker. He was diagnosed as hypothyroid ten years earlier and the only medication he is on is thyroxine 100μg daily. The staff say that he has taken this regularly until two days earlier and his records show that his thyroid function was checked six months earlier.

THYROID FUNCTION

	Result	Normal range
Thyroxine	125 nmol/l	70–140 nmol/l
Thyroid-stimulating hormone	1.6 mU/l	0.3–6.0 mU/l

On examination there is nothing abnormal to find apart from limitation of hip movement with pain and a little discomfort in the right loin.

INVESTIGATIONS AT THE RESIDENTIAL HOME

- Blood pressure   178/102
- Blood glucose   6.2 mmol/l
- Urine dipstick   negative for sugar, + for protein, + + for blood

The staff say that he is becoming demented and that the residential home is not an appropriate place for such patients.

QUESTION

- What should be done?

ANSWER 5

This is not the picture of dementia. The acute onset with clouding of consciousness, hallucinations, delusions, restlessness and disorientation suggest an **acute confusional state, delirium**. There are many causes of this state in the elderly. It can be provoked by drugs, infections, metabolic or endocrine disorders, or other underlying conditions in the heart, lungs, brain or abdomen.

There is no record of any drugs although this should be rechecked to rule out any analgesics or other agents that he might have had access to or might not be regarded as important.

In this case the thyroid abnormality is not likely to be relevant. The lack of replacement for 2 days will not have a significant effect and the normal results six months earlier make this an unlikely cause of his current problem. The sugar is normal. Other metabolic causes such as renal failure, anaemia, hyponatraemia and hypercalcaemia need to be excluded.

The falls raise the possibility of trauma and a subdural haematoma could present in this way. However, it seems that the falls were a secondary phenomenon. The most likely cause is that he has a urinary-tract infection. There is blood and protein in the urine, he has become incontinent and he has some tenderness in the loin which could fit with pyelonephritis. We are not told whether he had a fever and the white cell count should be measured.

If this does seem the likely diagnosis it would be best to treat him where he is if this is safe and possible. He is likely to be more confused by a move to a new environment in hospital. There is every likelihood that he will return to his previous state if the urinary-tract infection is confirmed and treated appropriately although this may take longer than the response in temperature and white cell count. Treatment should be started on the presumption of a urinary-tract infection while the diagnosis is confirmed by microscopy and culture of the urine. The most likely organism is *Escherichia coli* and an antibiotic such as trimethoprim would be appropriate, although resistance is possible and advice of the local microbiologist may be helpful.

✎ KEY POINTS

- Acute changes in mental state need to be explained even in the elderly with baseline mental problems.
- In delirium, consciousness is clouded, disorientation is usual and delusions may develop. The onset is acute. In dementia, there is an acquired global impairment of intellect, memory and personality, but consciousness is typically clear.

CASE 6

A 35-year-old man is seen in the casualty department because he has developed a painful, swollen right knee. This has occurred rapidly over the past 36 hours. There is no history of trauma to the knee or previous joint problems. He feels generally unwell and has also noticed his eyes to be sore. He has had no significant previous medical illnesses. He is married with two children. He is a non-smoker and drinks about 15 units of alcohol per week. He is a businessman and returned three weeks ago from a business trip to Thailand.

On examination, his temperature is 38.0°C. Both eyes appear red. There is a brown macular rash on his palms and soles. Examination of cardiovascular, respiratory, abdominal and neurological systems is normal. His right knee is swollen, hot and tender. No other joint appears to be affected.

INVESTIGATIONS

		Normal
Haemoglobin	13.8 g/dl	(13.3–17.7 g/dl)
Mean cell volume	87 fl	(80–99 fl)
White cell count	13.6 × 10⁹/l	(3.9–10.6 × 10⁹/l)
Platelets	345 × 10⁹/l	(150–440 × 10⁹/l)
Erythrocyte sedimentation rate	64 mm/h	(<10mm/h)
Sodium	139 mmol/l	(135–145 mmol/l)
Potassium	4.1 mmol/l	(3.5–5.0 mmol/l)
Urea	5.2 mmol/l	(2.5–6.7 mmol/l)
Creatinine	94 μmol/l	(70–120 μmol/l)
Urinalysis	no protein; no blood; no glucose	
Blood cultures	negative	
X-ray knee	soft-tissue swelling around joint	

QUESTIONS

- What is the diagnosis and what are the major differential diagnoses?
- How would you investigate and manage this patient?

ANSWER 6

This patient has a monoarthropathy, a rash and red eyes. Investigations show a raised white cell count and erythrocyte sedimentation rate (ESR). The diagnosis in this man was **Reiter's syndrome**. This disease classically presents with a triad of symptoms (although all three may not always be present):

- Seronegative arthritis affecting mainly lower limb joints
- Conjunctivitis
- Non-specific urethritis

Reiter's syndrome can be triggered by non-gonococcal urethritis (NGU) or by certain bowel infections. This patient is likely to have contracted NGU after sexual intercourse in Thailand. On direct questioning he admitted to the presence of an urethral discharge. The acute arthritis is typically a monoarthritis but can develop into a chronic relapsing destructive arthritis affecting the knees and feet and causing a sacroiliitis and spondylitis. Tendinitis and plantar fasciitis may occur. The red eyes are due to conjunctivitis and anterior uveitis and can recur with flares of the arthritis. The rash on the patient's palmar surfaces is the characteristic brown macular rash of this condition – keratoderma blenorrhagica. Other features of this condition that are sometimes seen include nail dystrophy and a circinate balanitis. Systemic manifestations such as pericarditis, pleuritis, fever and lymphadenopathy may occur in this disease. The ESR is usually elevated.

❗ DIFFERENTIAL DIAGNOSIS OF AN ACUTE MONOARTHRITIS

- Gonococcal arthritis (occasionally a polyarthritis affecting the small joints of the hands and wrists, with a pustular rash).
- Acute septic arthritis (the patient looks ill and septic and the skin over the joint is very erythematous).
- Other seronegative arthritides (ankylosing spondylitis, psoriatic arthropathy).
- Viral arthritis (usually polyarticular).
- Acute rheumatoid arthritis (usually polyarticular).
- Acute gout (most commonly affects the metatarsophalangeal joints).
- Pseudogout (caused by sodium pyrophosphate crystals; often affects large joints in older patients).
- Lyme disease (caused by *Borrelia burgdorfii* infection transmitted by a tick bite; may have the characteristic skin rash – erythema chronicum migrans).
- Haemorrhagic arthritis (usually a history of trauma or bleeding disorder).

This patient should have urethral swabs taken to exclude chlamydial/gonococcal infections and the appropriate antibiotics given. His knee should be aspirated. A Gram stain will exclude a pyogenic infection and birefringent microscopy used to detect uric acid or pyrophosphate crystals. This patient should be given non-steroidal anti-inflammatory drugs (NSAIDs) for the pain and he may require bed rest. If his disease relapses he should be referred to a rheumatologist. He and his wife should be referred to the sexually transmitted disease clinic for counselling and testing for other sexually transmitted diseases such as hepatitis B, HIV and syphilis.

A 32-year-old woman who lives alone calls the emergency general practitioner covering services at 2 am because of a 4-hour history of 'severe vomiting'. She has had very loose bowel motions on three occasions over the same period. There have been some cramping abdominal pains in the central and lower abdomen. These began 5–6 hours earlier. She smokes 10 cigarettes a day and drinks 3–4 glasses of wine 2–3 times a week. At lunchtime, she eats in the restaurant at work and cooks for herself most evenings. She is vegetarian. The previous evening there had been an office party at which she had eaten prawn sandwiches, egg mayonnaise and profiteroles.

There has been no dysuria. Her periods have always been rather irregular and the last menstrual period was five weeks ago.

She does not take any regular medication. She works as a secretary in an accountancy firm. She has two cats. She was on holiday in Spain six weeks earlier. In her previous medical history she had an appendicectomy ten years ago. She had a termination of pregnancy 12 years previously. In the family history, her father has maturity-onset diabetes mellitus.

On examination, she is lying in bed and looks unwell. Her temperature is 38.0°C. She does not look anaemic. Her pulse is 104/min and regular. The blood pressure is 108/62. Her respiratory rate is 20/min. Her tongue looks dry. She has some tenderness in the centre of the abdomen and in the left iliac fossa. There is no guarding. The hernial orifices are normal. On listening to her abdomen, the bowel sounds are prominent. There is no lymphadenopathy.

Dipstick testing of her urine shows no protein, sugar or blood but a trace of ketones.

She says that this is a very busy time at the office and wants to have some treatment so that she will be able to go to work the next day.

QUESTIONS

- What is the likely diagnosis?
- What should be done?

ANSWER 7

The sudden onset of diarrhoea and vomiting sounds most like an episode of **acute infective gastroenteritis**. There is no evidence of peritoneal irritation to suggest a more serious local pathology in the abdomen. The sudden onset and the presence of diarrhoea makes other diagnoses such as pregnancy unlikely although it would be worth checking a pregnancy test since it is five weeks since her last period.

The commonest causes of infective gastroenteritis in the United Kingdom are viruses such as rotaviruses, *Campylobacter jejuni* and *Salmonella enteritidis*. Other organisms such as *Staphylococcus* or *Escherichia coli* food poisoning are also possible. It seems possible that the office lunch might be the source of the problem in which case *Salmonella* is the more likely bacterial pathogen since the source is often eggs or dairy products and the incubation period 8–48 hours compared to 2–4 days for *Campylobacter*.

The initial decision that needs to be made is whether there is significant dehydration already and whether she is going to be able to maintain her hydration at home in the presence of diarrhoea and vomiting. The finding of a trace of ketones in the urine is common in patients unable to eat for some hours. There is no sugar in the urine and the family history of non-insulin-dependent diabetes is not likely to be relevant. Her pulse rate is fast and her blood pressure rather low although it may be normal for her. The blood pressure should be measured lying and standing to see if there is a postural drop suggesting intravascular dehydration.

Since she lives alone and the diarrhoea and vomiting are severe it would be safer to admit her to hospital where she can be rehydrated intravenously. Her vomiting could be treated with an anti-emetic which would be more likely to be effective if it were given intramuscularly or intravenously in view of her vomiting. It is not usually necessary to treat the diarrhoea symptomatically in this situation but just to replace the fluid loss. An antibiotic such as the quinolone ciprofloxacin can be used and may shorten the period of diarrhoea in bacterial enteritis without increasing the chronic carriage of *Salmonella*. However, such episodes can usually be managed simply by maintaining adequate fluid replacement.

Electrolytes, urea and creatinine should be measured. Liver-function tests, full blood picture and amylase to rule out pancreatitis would be useful. Stool should be sent for culture since *Salmonella* infection is a notifiable disease in the United Kingdom. Blood cultures may be positive.

KEY POINTS

- 'Food poisoning' is a notifiable disease in the United Kingdom.
- The major element of management of infective gastroenteritis is maintenance of hydration with oral or intravenous fluids.

CASE 8

A 21-year-old man is brought in to hospital at 5 pm. He was found unconscious at home in his flat by his girlfriend. She had last seen him at 8 pm the evening before when they came home after Christmas shopping. When she came around the next afternoon she found him unconscious on the floor of the bathroom. There was no sign of any trauma or any drugs. He had been well previously with no known medical history. There was a family history of diabetes mellitus in his father and one of his two brothers.

His girlfriend had said that he had shown no signs of unusual mood on the previous day. He had his end of term examinations in psychology coming up in one week and was anxious about these but his studies seemed to be going well and there had been no problems with previous examinations.

On examination he looked pale. His pulse was 92/min, blood pressure 114/74, respiratory rate 22/min. There were no abnormalities to find in the cardiovascular or respiratory systems. In the nervous system there was no response to verbal commands. Appropriate withdrawal movements were made in response to pain. The reflexes were brisk and symmetrical, plantars were downgoing. In the fundi, the optic disks appeared swollen.

QUESTION

- What are the most likely diagnoses and what other investigations should be done immediately?

ANSWER 8

This young man has been brought in unconscious having been well less than 24 hours previously. The most likely diagnoses are related to drugs or a neurological event. The first part of the care should be to ensure that he is stable from a cardiac and respiratory point of view. His respiratory rate is a little high. Blood gases should be measured to monitor the oxygenation and ensure that the carbon dioxide level is not high, suggesting hypoventilation.

The family history of diabetes raises the possibility that his problem is related to this. However, the speed of onset makes hyperglycaemic coma unlikely. One would expect the slower development with a history of thirst and polyuria over the last day or so. However, the blood sugar should certainly be checked. Hypoglycaemia comes on faster but would not occur as a new event in diabetes mellitus. It might occur as a manifestation of a rare condition such as an insulinoma. Other metabolic causes of coma such as abnormal levels of sodium or calcium should be checked.

A neurological problem such as a subarachnoid haemorrhage is possible as a sudden unexpected event in a young person. Where the level of consciousness is so affected some localizing signs or subhyaloid haemorrhage in the fundi might be expected. If no other cause is evident from the initial investigations, a computed tomography (CT) scan might be indicated.

The most likely cause is that the loss of consciousness is drug related. Despite the lack of any warning of intent beforehand, drug overdose is common and the question of availability of any medication should be explored further. This would be likely to be a sedative drug. If there is any suspicion of this then levels of other drugs which might need treatment should be measured, e.g. aspirin and paracetamol.

The other possibility in somebody brought in unconscious is **carbon monoxide poisoning**. The fact that it is winter and he was found in the bathroom where a faulty gas-fired heater might be situated increases this possibility. Patients with carbon monoxide poisoning are usually pale rather than the traditional cherry-red colour associated with carboxyhaemoglobin. Papilloedema can occur in severe carbon monoxide poisoning and might account for the swollen appearance of the optic disks on fundoscopy.

Measurement of carboxyhaemoglobin showed a level of 32 per cent. He was treated with high levels of inspired oxygen and made a slow but full recovery over the next 48 hours. The problem was traced to a faulty gas water heater which had not been serviced for four years.

KEY POINTS

- Drug overdose is the commonest cause of unconsciousness in young people but other diagnoses must always be considered.
- Carboxyhaemoglobin levels should be measured in patients found unconscious indoors or in vehicles and after known exposure to smoke.

CASE 9

A 44-year-old man is referred to a hypertension clinic by his GP. His hypertension is newly diagnosed having been detected at a routine medical. His blood pressure has been around 170/110 and has not been easily controlled. The GP organizes blood tests which show marked hypokalaemia. He also complains of thirst and polyuria, as well as general weakness and muscle cramps. There is no significant past medical history. There is no family history of renal disease or hypertension. He is a lorry driver, smokes 20 cigarettes per day and drinks 25 units of alcohol per week. He is on nifedipine 20 mg twice daily.

On examination he looks well. His pulse is 84/min regular, blood pressure 170/112, jugular venous pressure not raised, heart sounds normal. Examination of the respiratory, abdominal and neurological systems is normal. Fundoscopy shows arteriovenous nipping and silver wiring.

INVESTIGATIONS

		Normal
Haemoglobin	13.4 g/dl	(13.3–17.7 g/dl)
White cell count	4.2×10^9/l	($3.9–10.6 \times 10^9$/l)
Platelets	156×10^9/l	($150–440 \times 10^9$/l)
Sodium	147 mmol/l	(135–145 mmol/l)
Potassium	2.2 mmol/l	(3.5–5.0 mmol/l)
Bicarbonate	32 mmol/l	(24–30 mmol/l)
Urea	3.9 mmol/l	(2.5–6.7 mmol/l)
Creatinine	84 μmol/l	(70–120 μmol/l)
Glucose	5.6 mmol/l	(4.0–6.0 mmol/l)
Urinalysis	no protein; no blood	
24-h urinary potassium excretion	50 mmol	(40–120 mmol/24 h)
ECG	sinus rhythm; flattened T-waves in all leads	
Renal ultrasound	two normal-sized kidneys	

QUESTIONS

- What is the underlying diagnosis in this patient?
- How would you investigate and manage this patient?

ANSWER 9

This patient has severe hypokalaemia (with an associated metabolic alkalosis shown by the raised bicarbonate). Severe hypokalaemia causes muscle weakness, paralytic ileus and cardiac arrythmias. ECG changes include flattening of the T-wave, depression of the ST segment and prominent U-waves.

! CAUSES OF HYPOKALAEMIA

• Gastrointestinal losses	diarrhoea/vomiting; ileostomy
• Urinary losses	diuretics
	secondary hyperaldosteronism
	glucocorticoid excess (Cushing's disease)
	primary hyperaldosteronism
	liquorice to excess
	rare renal tubular defects, e.g. renal tubular acidosis, or genetic defects of transporter proteins, e.g. Liddle's, Bartter's or Gitelman's syndrome
• Redistribution	metabolic alkalosis; insulin/glucose treatment hypokalaemic periodic paralysis
• Decreased intake	chronic starvation

The combination of hypertension, hypokalaemia and alkalosis, without clinical or biochemical features of glucocorticoid excess make **primary hyperaldosteronism** the most likely diagnosis. A plasma sodium in the higher part of the reference range due to sodium retention and a 24-hour urinary potassium excretion > 30mmol/l despite serum hypokalaemia are characteristic.

To confirm the diagnosis of primary hyperaldosteronism, a low plasma renin activity should be found in the presence of a high plasma aldosterone level. In contrast, in accelerated hypertension, renovascular disease and diuretic-induced hypokalaemia high renin levels will be found. The commonest causes of primary hyperaldosteronism are adrenal adenomas and adrenal hyperplasia. Computed tomography (CT) scanning will visualize the adrenals (Fig. 9.1 shows a right adrenal tumour (arrow) adjacent to the liver). Selective adrenal vein catheterization or nuclear medicine scanning provides functional data. Figure 9.2 shows an adrenal scintiscan (using [75] Se-cholesterol) in a different patient with bilateral adrenal hyperplasia; a gamma camera picture on day 10 after intravenous injection shows bilateral uptake (arrows). Aldosterone-secreting adenomas should be treated surgically, with cure of hypertension in about 50 per cent of cases. Idiopathic hyperaldosteronism should be treated with spironolactone and glucocorticoid-remediable hyperaldosteronism with dexamethasone.

🔑 KEY POINT

• Common causes of hypertension and hypokalaemia include diuretic-treated hypertension, renovascular disease and accelerated hypertension and, more rarely, primary hyperaldosteronism.

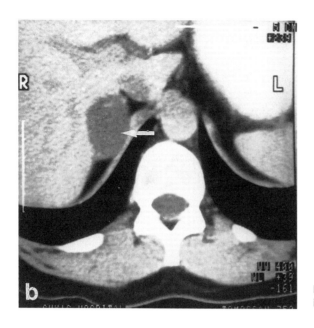

Figure 9.1 CT scan show-ing right adrenal tumor

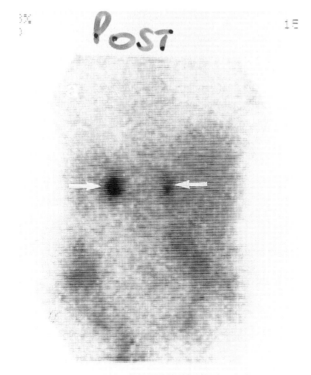

Figure 9.2 Adrenal scintis-can showing bilateral adrenal hyperplasia

CASE 10

A 23-year-old woman presents to her GP complaining that she has recently developed multiple spontaneous bruises over her trunk and limbs, and has been having an exceptionally heavy period. She feels extremely tired and has been off work for the past week. She has also noted a painful ulcer on her palate which is not healing. She has no past history of easy bruising and has had previous dental extractions without incident. She has had no significant previous medical illnesses. There is no family history of a bleeding abnormality. She works as a nurse. She is a non-smoker and drinks about 15 units of alcohol per week.

On examination her conjunctivae are pale. There are multiple bruises over her limbs and trunk. There is a deep ulcer on her soft palate with oral *Candida* present. Her gums are bleeding spontaneously. There is no lymphadenopathy. Fundoscopy reveals retinal haemorrhages. Examination is otherwise normal.

BLOOD TESTS

		Normal
Haemoglobin	6.2 g/dl	(11.7–15.7 g/dl)
Mean cell volume	89 fl	(80–99 fl)
White cell count	1.2×10^9/l	$(3.5–11.0 \times 10^9$/l)
Neutrophils	0.2×10^9/l	$(1.8–7.7 \times 10^9$/l)
Eosinophils	0.1×10^9/l	$(0.20 \times 10^9$/l)
Lymphocytes	0.7×10^9/l	$(1.0–4.8 \times 10^9$/l)
Monocytes	0.1×10^9/l	$(0–0.8 \times 10^9$/l)
Blood film	small number of blast cells present	
Platelets	8×10^9/l	$(150–440 \times 10^9$/l)
Erythrocyte sedimentation rate	15 mm/h	(<10 mm/h)
Sodium	138 mmol/l	(135–145 mmol/l)
Potassium	4.2 mmol/l	(3.5–5.0 mmol/l)
Urea	6.4 mmol/l	(2.5–6.7 mmol/l)
Creatinine	106 μmol/l	(70–120 μmol/l)
Glucose	4.8 mmol/l	(4.0–6.0 mmol/l)
Prothrombin time		normal
Activated partial thromboplastin time		normal

QUESTIONS

- What is the likely diagnosis?
- What are the major differential diagnoses?
- How would you investigate and manage this patient?

ANSWER 10

This woman is pancytopenic with anaemia, leukopenia and thrombocytopenia.

The blood film appearance of immature blast cells indicates a diagnosis of **acute leukaemia**. This patient is tired because of her severe anaemia. Mouth ulceration due to herpes simplex virus and *Candida* infection is common in profoundly neutropenic patients. Her major presenting complaint is with a severe bleeding tendency due to her thrombocytopenia. An abnormal bleeding tendency may be due to platelet, coagulation or blood vessel abnormalities. Platelet/vessel defects cause purpura in the skin and mucous membranes often unrelated to trauma, but with immediate bleeding following trauma. Coagulation defects cause haematomas and haemarthroses often in response to trauma but usually with a time delay after the trauma. A positive family history or early age of onset of bleeding suggests haemophilia. On examination, the distribution of bruising may be diagnostic. Thrombocytopenic purpura is usually seen over pressure areas and dependent areas (ankles). Senile purpura and steroid-induced bruising characteristically occur on the forearms and backs of the hands. Henoch–Schönlein purpura occurs over the extensor surfaces of the limbs and buttocks. The combination of thrombocytopenia and anaemia may lead to retinal haemorrhages.

This woman needs urgent referral to a haematology unit. A bone-marrow aspiration and trephine biopsy will reveal abnormal blasts which can be characterized morphologically, immunologically with monoclonal antibodies and genetically (using the polymerase chain reaction) to precisely classify the type of acute leukaemia.

Once a diagnosis is established, the prognosis and treatment should be discussed with the patient and family. The patient will be treated with chemotherapy and possibly bone-marrow transplantation. She should be advised to contact the unit immediately she develops a fever because of the risks of overwhelming septicaemia in a neutropenic patient.

⚲ KEY POINTS

- Purpura is usually due to thrombocytopenia or vessel-wall disorders, whereas haematomas reflect clotting factor defects.
- Visceral bleeding, heavy menstrual bleeding or recurrent nosebleeds may be clues that a bleeding disorder is present.

A 38-year-old woman presents to a casualty department complaining of a severe headache. The headache started 24 hours previously and has rapidly become more intense. It is generalized and associated with vomiting, drowsiness and confusion. She is unable to tolerate being in a bright room. She has no significant medical history. She smokes 20 cigarettes per day and drinks 15 units of alcohol per week. She is on no medication. She does not work and has two children aged six and eight years.

On examination, she looks flushed and unwell. Her temperature is 39.0°C. Her neck is stiff and it is painful to move her head. There is no rash. Her sinuses are not tender and her eardrums appear normal. Her pulse rate is 124/min and blood pressure 94/72. Examination of heart, chest and abdomen are normal. Her conscious level is decreased but she is rousable to command and she has no focal neurological signs. Her fundi are normal.

INVESTIGATIONS

		Normal
Haemoglobin	12.2 g/dl	(11.7–15.7 g/dl)
White cell count	18.4 × 10⁹/l	(3.5–11.0 × 10⁹/l)
Platelets	322 × 10⁹/l	(150–440 × 10⁹/l)
Sodium	129 mmol/l	(135–145 mmol/l)
Potassium	3.7 mmol/l	(3.5–5.0 mmol/l)
Urea	12.4 mmol/l	(2.5–6.7 mmol/l)
Creatinine	186 μmol/l	(70–120 μmol/l)
Glucose	5.8 mmol/l	(4.0–6.0 mmol/l)
Blood cultures	results awaited	
Chest X-ray	normal	
ECG	sinus tachycardia	
CT brain	normal	
Lumbar puncture	turbid CSF	
Leukocytes	> 8000/μl	(< 5 ml)
CSF protein	1.4 g/l	(< 0.4 g/l)
CSF glucose	0.8 mmol/l	(> 70 per cent plasma glucose)
Gram stain	result awaited	

QUESTIONS

- What is the diagnosis?
- What are the major differential diagnoses?
- How would you manage this patient?

ANSWER 11

This patient has **bacterial meningitis**. She has presented with sudden onset of severe headache, vomiting, confusion, photophobia and neck stiffness. The presence of hypotension, leukocytosis and renal impairment suggest acute bacterial infection rather than viral meningitis. The most likely causative organisms are *Neisseria meningitidis*, *Haemophilus influenzae* and *Streptococcus pneumonia*. In patients in this age group the last is the most likely organism. Meningococcal meningitis is usually associated with a generalized vasculitic rash.

The most severe headaches are experienced in meningitis, subarachnoid haemorrhage and classic migraine. Meningitis, subarachnoid haemorrhage and temporal arteritis present as single episodes of headaches. Meningitis usually presents over hours whereas subarachnoid haemorrhage presents very suddenly. Fundoscopy in patients with subarachnoid haemorrhage may show subhyaloid haemorrhage. Meningeal irritation is seen in many acute febrile conditions especially in children and local infections of the neck/spine may cause neck stiffness. Other causes of meningitis include viral, fungal, cryptococcal and tuberculous meningitis which can be distinguished by analysis of the CSF.

Patients with no papilloedema or lateralizing neurological signs that suggest a space-occupying lesion should be lumbar punctured immediately (even before a CT scan is obtained). The combination of >1000 neutrophils/μl CSF, a CSF glucose <40 per cent of the simultaneous blood level and a CSF protein > 1.5 g/l is strongly suggestive of bacterial meningitis. The Gram stain and culture will give the definitive diagnosis. In this case, the Gram stain demonstrated Gram-positive cocci consistent with *Streptococcus pneumonia* infection. Intravenous antibiotics must be started immediately. The patient must be nursed in a manner appropriate for the decreased conscious level. Adequate analgesia with opiates should be given. The patient has mild hyponatraemia due to the syndrome of inappropriate antidiuretic hormone (ADH) secretion, and fluid losses should be treated with normal saline. Inotropes may be needed to treat hypotension.

The two children aged six and eight years must be considered. It is not clear from the history who is looking after them. They should be examined and if meningococcal meningitis is suspected or the organism is uncertain they should be given prophylactic treatment with rifampicin and vaccinated against meningococcal meningitis.

♀ KEY POINTS

- Bacterial meningitis causes severe headache, neck stiffness, drowsiness and photophobia.
- The main differential diagnoses are subarachnoid haemorrhage and migraine.

A 34-year-old woman presents to her GP complaining of a rash. Over the past two weeks she has developed multiple tender red swellings on her shins and forearms. The older swellings are darker in colour and seem to be healing from the centre. She feels generally unwell and tired and also has pains in her wrists and ankles. The woman has not had a recent sore throat. Over the past two years she has had recurrent aphthous ulcers in her mouth and has had intermittent abdominal pain and diarrhoea. She works as a waitress and is unmarried. She smokes about 15 cigarettes per day and drinks alcohol only occasionally. She has had no previous medical illnesses.

On examination there are multiple tender lesions on the shins and forearms. The lesions are raised and vary from 1 to 3 cm in diameter. The fresher lesions are red and the older ones look like bruises. She is thin but looks well. Physical examination is otherwise normal.

INVESTIGATIONS

		Normal
Haemoglobin	13.5 g/dl	(11.7–15.7 g/dl)
White cell count	15.4 × 10⁹/l	(3.5–11.0 × 10⁹/l)
Platelets	198 × 10⁹/l	(150–440 × 10⁹/l)
Erythrocyte sedimentation rate	98 mm/hr	(< 10mm/hr)
Sodium	138 mmol/l	(135–145 mmol/l)
Potassium	4.3 mmol/l	(3.5–5.0 mmol/l)
Urea	5.4 mmol/l	(2.5–6.7 mmol/l)
Creatinine	86 μmol/l	(70–120 μmol/l)
Glucose	5.8 mmol/l	(4.0–6.0 mmol/l)
Chest X-ray	normal	
Urinalysis	normal	

QUESTIONS

- What is the diagnosis?
- What are the major causes of this condition?

ANSWER 12

This patient has **erythema nodosum**, in this case secondary to previously undiagnosed Crohn's disease. Erythema nodosum is due to inflammation of the small blood vessels in the deep dermis. Characteristically it affects the shins, but it may also affect the thighs and forearms. The number and size of the lesions is variable. Lesions tend to heal from the centre and spread peripherally. The rash is often preceded by systemic symptoms – fever, malaise and arthralgia. It usually resolves over 3–4 weeks, but persistence or recurrence suggests an underlying disease.

! DISEASES LINKED TO ERYTHEMA NODOSUM

- Streptococcal infection
- Tuberculosis
- Leprosy
- Glandular fever
- Histoplasmosis
- Coccidioidomycosis
- Lymphoma/leukaemia
- Sarcoidosis
- Pregnancy/oral contraceptive
- Sulphonamides
- Ulcerative colitis
- Crohn's disease

The history of mouth ulcers, abdominal pain and diarrhoea strongly suggests that this woman has Crohn's disease. She should therefore be referred to a gastroenterologist for investigations which should include a small bowel enema and colonoscopy with biopsies. Treatment of her underlying disease with steroids should cause the erythema nodosum to resolve. With no serious underlying condition erythema nodosum usually settles with non-steroidal anti-inflammatory drugs.

⚲ KEY POINTS

- Patients presenting with erythema nodosum should be investigated for an underlying disease.
- Erythema nodosum is most often seen on the shins but can affect the extensor surface of the forearms or thighs.

CASE 13

A 60-year-old woman attends her GP's surgery complaining of breathlessness on exertion. This had been increasing over the last eight months until it is now producing problems at around 500 yards walking on the level or a flight of stairs. On two or three occasions she has woken at night with mild shortness of breath. There was no history of chest pain. She has had several bouts of fast palpitations which lasted 20–30 min and were a little distressing and associated with some shortness of breath. These episodes of palpitations had occurred at rest; she was unclear about the rate or the rhythm but thought that they were probably irregular. Occasionally, her ankles become swollen by the end of the day but go down again overnight.

She smokes 10 cigarettes each day and drinks 10 units of alcohol each week. She is on no medication. In her previous medical history she had a hysterectomy for fibroids ten years previously. There is a family history of asthma; two of her four brothers and one of her two children have had mild asthma. She worked as a cleaner part-time but gave this up three months previously because of the breathlessness. She eats well and complains of no other symptoms on direct questioning.

Initial observations show a regular pulse of 80/min and a blood pressure of 110/72. Her chest X-ray is shown in Fig.13.1.

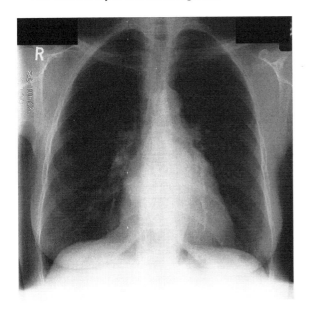

Figure 13.1

QUESTION

- What would you expect to find on examination of the cardiovascular and respiratory systems?

ANSWER 13

The chest X-ray shows a normal sized heart but a prominent bulge high up on the left border of the heart which is consistent with an enlarged left atrial appendage. There is no evidence of pulmonary oedema on the chest X-ray. This would be consistent with a diagnosis of pure **mitral stenosis**, the increased pressure in the left atrium causing it to dilate. Mitral regurgitation would produce volume overload of the left ventricle also with dilatation and enlargement of the cardiac diameter on the X-ray.

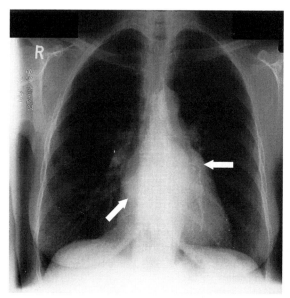

There is a family history of asthma and peak expiratory flow should be measured to exclude an element of asthma. The term 'cardiac asthma' was used for pulmonary oedema in the past because shortness of breath may be intermittent and wheezing may be heard. In this case, the findings indicate a different cause for the symptoms.

Mitral stenosis would produce a loud first heart sound, an opening snap followed by a rumbling mid-diastolic murmur with a presystolic crescendo at the time of atrial contraction since she is in sinus rhythm. On listening to the chest, there

Figure 13.1 X-ray of normal size heart with enlarged left atrium (arrowed)

might be some late inspiratory crackles to hear at the lung bases. On examination, a prominent localized pulsation at the apex and a prominent first heart sound would be early clues. The patient should be turned to the left side to hear the murmur better using the bell of the stethoscope and exercising her gently if it remains difficult to hear.

The palpitations are likely to be episodes of atrial fibrillation related to disruption of normal conduction in the dilated left atrium. Echocardiography would confirm the diagnosis of mitral stenosis and give an assessment of the severity and any associated findings. The term 'palpitations' needs to be interpreted with care since patients may have different ideas about what is meant. The patient's precise meaning should be explored. It is not unusual for patients to find it difficult to describe the pattern of the arrhythmia precisely. Sometimes getting them to tap out the rhythm of the heartbeat can be helpful.

In this case, echocardiography confirmed the diagnosis. The rhythm settled in to atrial fibrillation needing digoxin to control the rate and warfarin to reduce the risk of systemic emboli. Mitral valvuloplasty was used to reduce the severity of the mitral stenosis.

- Pure mitral stenosis enlarges the left atrium but does not cause enlargement of the left ventricle or displacement of the apex beat.
- Asking patients to tap out the rhythm or tapping out options for them may help to explore the meaning of the symptom of palpitations.

CASE 14

A 75-year-old widow has been feeling unwell with upper abdominal pain. The pain has increased over the last 4 days. It has been a general ache in the upper abdomen with some more severe waves of pain. She has vomited four times. On two or three occasions in the past four years she has had a more severe pain in the right upper abdomen. This has sometimes been associated with fever and was treated with antibiotics on one occasion. Her appetite has been good until the last week when she has been off her food. She has not lost any weight. She has had no urinary or bowel problems but comments that her urine has been darker than usual for a few days.

In her previous medical history she has had hypothyroidism and is on replacement thyroxine. She has annual blood tests to check on the dose; the last test was two months ago. She has had some episodes of chest pain on exercise once or twice a week for six months and has been given atenolol 50 mg daily and a glyceryl trinitrate spray to use sublingually as needed.

On examination, her sclerae are yellow. Her pulse is 56/min and regular. Her blood pressure is 124/82. There are no abnormalities in the cardiovascular system or respiratory system. She is tender in the right upper abdomen. No masses are palpable in the abdomen. She is clinically euthyroid.

INVESTIGATIONS

		Normal
Sodium	140 mmol/l	(135–145 mmol/l)
Potassium	4.0 mmol/l	(3.5–5.0 mmol/l)
Urea	6.6 mmol/l	(2.5–6.7 mmol/l)
Creatinine	112 μmol/l	(70–120 μmol/l)
Calcium	2.44 mmol/l	(2.12–2.65 mmol/l)
Phosphate	1.19 mmol/l	(0.8–1.45 mmol/l)
Total bilirubin	88 μmol/l	(3–17 μmol/l)
Alkaline phosphatase	942 IU/l	(30–300 IU/l)
Alanine aminotransferase	54 IU/l	(5–35 IU/l)
Gamma-glutamyl transpeptidase	468 IU/l	(11–51 IU/l)
Thyroid-stimulating hormone	1.8 mU/l	(0.3–6.0 mU/l)

QUESTIONS

- How do you interpret these findings?
- What is the appropriate management?

ANSWER 14

This woman has a four-year history of intermittent upper abdominal pain. Her current pain has lasted longer than previous episodes and on examination she is jaundiced.

Her investigations show a raised bilirubin. The alanine aminotransferase is slightly raised but the main abnormalities in the liver enzymes are in alkaline phosphatase and gamma-glutamyl transpeptidase. This is the pattern of **obstructive jaundice** which can be caused by mechanical obstruction by tumour or by gallstones, or by adverse effects of some drugs (e.g. phenothiazines, flucloxacillin). The drugs she is taking are not likely causes of liver problems.

The previous episodes of pain and fever over the last four years are likely to have been cholecystitis secondary to gallstones. If the gallbladder were to be palpable on examination this would suggest an alternative diagnosis of malignant obstruction since by this time these previous episodes of cholecystitis would usually have caused scarring and contraction of the gallbladder. In order to produce obstructive jaundice one or more of her gallstones must have moved out of the gallbladder and impacted in the common bile duct. Migration of gallstones from the gallbladder occurs in around 15 per cent of cases.

Her thyroid condition seems to be stable and not relevant to the current problem. Her angina is indicative of coronary artery disease and needs to be considered when treatment is being planned for her gallstones.

Only a minority of gallstones are radio-opaque and visible on a plain radiograph so the next investigation should be an ultrasound of the liver and biliary tract. Ultrasound will show dilatation of the biliary tree but is not so reliable for identifying common bile duct stones. Endoscopic retrograde cholangiopancreatography (ERCP) is the best tool for this and sphincterotomy with or without stone retrieval may be possible to remove stones obstructing the common bile duct.

KEY POINTS

- Obstructive jaundice with a dilated, palpable gallbladder is likely to be caused by carcinoma at the head of the pancreas (Courvoisier's sign).
- Obstructive jaundice causes preferential elevation of alkaline phosphatase and gamma-glutamyl transpeptidase. When the main rise is in alanine aminotransferase, this indicates primarily hepatocellular damage.

CASE 15

A 64-year-old woman has a ten-year history of retrosternal pain. The pain is often present in bed at night and may be precipitated by bending down. Occasionally, the pain comes on after eating and on some occasions it appears to have been precipitated by exercise. The pain has been described as having a burning and a tight quality to it. The pain is not otherwise exacerbated by respiratory movements or position.

Her husband has angina and on one occasion she took one of his glyceryl trinitrate tablets. She thinks that this probably helped her pain since it seemed to go off a little faster than usual. She has also bought some indigestion tablets from a local pharmacy and thinks that these probably helped also.

On examination she is 5 feet 4 inches tall (1.62 m) and weighs 82 kg. There are no abnormalities to find in cardiovascular, respiratory or gastrointestinal systems.

Her chest X-ray is normal and the electrocardiogram is shown in Fig. 15.1. She had an exercise ECG performed and she was able to perform 8-min exercise. Her heart rate went up to 130/min with no change in the ST segments on the ECG and normal heart and blood-pressure responses. The haemoglobin, renal and liver function are normal.

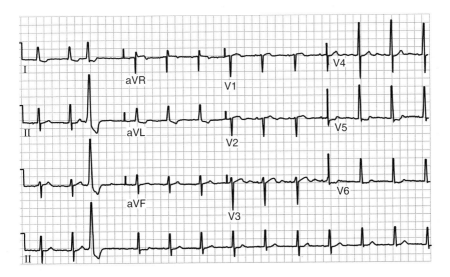

Figure 15.1

QUESTION

- What is the likely diagnosis and what would be appropriate management?

ANSWER 15

A number of features in the history make **oesophageal reflux** a likely diagnosis. The character and position of the pain and the relation to lying flat and to bending mean reflux is more likely. She is overweight, increasing the likelihood of reflux. The improvement with glyceryl trinitrate and with proprietary antacids is inconclusive. The ECG shows one ventricular ectopic and some T-wave changes in leads I, aVl, V5 and V6 which would be compatible with myocardial ischaemia but are not specific. The exercise ECG was negative which reduces the likelihood of ischaemic heart disease although it certainly does not rule it out. Other causes of chest pain are less likely with the length of history.

In view of the long history and the features suggesting oesophageal reflux, it would be reasonable to initiate a trial of therapy for oesophageal reflux with regular antacid therapy, H$_2$-receptor blockers or a proton pump inhibitor (omeprazole or lansoprazole). If the pain responds to this form of therapy, then additional actions such as weight loss (she is well above ideal body weight) and raising the head of the bed at night should be added. If doubt remains, a barium swallow should show the tendency to reflux and a gastroscopy would show evidence of oesophagitis. There is a broad association between the presence of oesophageal reflux, evidence of oesophagitis at endoscopy and biopsy, and the symptoms of heart burn. However, each can occur independently of the others.

Recording of pH in the oesophagus over 24 hours can provide additional useful information. It is achieved by passing a small pH-sensitive electrode into the oesophagus through the nose. This provides an objective measure of the amount of acid reaching the oesophagus and the times when this occurs.

This woman had an endoscopy which showed oesophagitis and treatment with omeprazole and an alginate relieved her symptoms. Attempts at weight loss were not successful.

KEY POINTS

- In non-specific chest pain with a normal ECG, the oesophagus is a common source of the pain.
- 24-hour pH recording in the oesophagus provides further information on acid reflux.

CASE 16

A 40-year-old farmer developed a fever and rigors. Over the next 6 hours he developed a dry cough and he also complains of some upper abdominal pain. He felt progressively more unwell and is brought to the accident & emergency department. He had been well previously with no significant medical history. There is no relevant family history. His farm is a small dairy farm that he manages with his wife and 18-year-old son.

On examination, he has a temperature of 39°C, a pulse rate of 104/min and a blood pressure of 120/82. The respiratory rate is 30/min. On examination of the chest, the trachea and apex beat are not displaced. There is dullness to percussion anteriorly on the right side. There is increased tactile vocal fremitus anteromedially on the right and in the right axilla, and the breath sounds are bronchial in the same area. In the abdomen, he has mild tenderness in the upper abdomen. There is no guarding and the bowel sounds are normal.

The chest X-ray is shown in Fig.16.1.

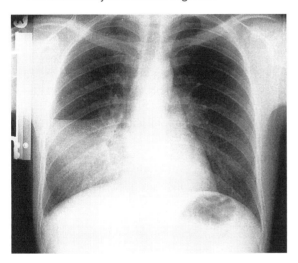

Figure 16.1

QUESTIONS

- What is the likely diagnosis?
- What would be the appropriate initial treatment?

ANSWER 16

The signs of dullness, increased tactile vocal fremitus and bronchial breathing without mediastinal shift are those of consolidation. The distribution anteriorly on the right and into the axilla place the consolidation in the middle lobe. These signs fit with the X-ray changes which show a straight upper border to the consolidation produced by the transverse fissure. An air bronchogram within the shadowing is the characteristic X-ray appearance of consolidation. Abdominal pain is a common symptom of pneumonia, more particularly when it involves the lower lobe which has greatest contact with the diaphragm. The tenderness in the upper abdomen may be related to the coughing.

His occupation raises the possibility of conditions such as extrinsic allergic alveolitis (farmer's lung) and the symptoms of fever, rigors and dry cough would fit this diagnosis. However, the local findings in the right lung show that there is a localized rather than a generalized problem in the lungs. These are the findings of lobar pneumonia. This is a **community acquired pneumonia** with no known underlying illness and the commonest cause is *Streptococcus pneumoniae* (ca. 50 per cent) which would fit well with the acute onset with fever and rigors. His occupation increases the chances of less common conditions such as legionellosis, Q fever or even leptospirosis.

In a moderately ill patient with pneumonia, a reasonable starting treatment would be intravenous cefuroxime and erythromycin. If there was a strong suspicion that the cause was *Streptococcus pneumoniae* in a previously fit patient, more targeted therapy such as benzylpenicillin would be reasonable as initial treatment. In some countries, penicillin resistance is emerging as an important factor in relation to *Streptococcus pneumoniae*.

In this case, pneumococci were isolated from the blood culture taken at admission. The erythromycin which had been part of the starting treatment in case of atypical organisms such as *legionella* was stopped and he made a good recovery with the cephalosporin antibiotic.

🔍 KEY POINTS

- An air bronchogram and anatomically defined distribution are the characteristic radiographic features of lobar pneumonia.
- Abdominal pain may be a feature of pneumonia, especially when a lower lobe is involved.

A 32-year-old man presents to his GP with a fever and general aching. At first he thought that this was probably influenza but the symptoms have now been present for 8 or 9 days. He has had aches in the muscles around the back and the legs. For 3 days he had diarrhoea but this has settled now. He has complained of a sore mouth which has made it difficult to eat but he has not felt very hungry during this time and thinks he may have lost a few kilograms in weight. He had noticed a mild erythematous rash over the trunk but this had faded.

He has visited the practice occasionally in the past for minor complaints. Six months earlier he became anxious because a friend had been found to be positive on testing for HIV. The friend is well and they had not seen each other for a year. The patient was tested and found to be negative. He smokes 10 cigarettes daily, drinks 20–30 units of alcohol weekly and takes no illicit drugs. He had no other relevant medical or family history. He works as a solicitor. He is single and lives alone. He has had a number of heterosexual and homosexual relationships in the past. He had not travelled outside the UK in the last year.

On examination, he had a temperature of 38°C. Pulse rate was 90/min, respiratory rate 16/min and blood pressure 118/76. There were no abnormalities in the cardio-vascular or respiratory system. On examination of the mouth there were two ulcers in the mucosa, 5–10 mm in diameter. There were a number of enlarged cervical lymph nodes which were a little tender. There were no rashes on the skin.

INVESTIGATIONS

		Normal
Haemoglobin	14.9 g/dl	13.7–17.7 g/dl
Mean corpuscular volume (MCV)	88 fl	80.5–99.7 fl
White cell count	6.4×10^9/l	$3.9–10.6 \times 10^9$/l
Neutrophils	4.1×10^9/l	$1.8–7.7 \times 10^9$/l
Lymphocytes	2.0×10^9/l	$0.6–4.8 \times 10^9$/l
Platelet count	316×10^9/l	$150–440 \times 10^9$/l
Sodium	145 mmol/l	135–145 mmol/l
Potassium	4.5 mmol/l	3.5–5.0 mmol/l
Urea	6.1 mmol/l	2.5–6.7 mmol/l
Creatinine	75 μmol/l	70–120 μmol/l
Bilirubin	14 μmol/l	3–17 μmol/l
Alkaline phosphatase	101 IU/l	30–300 IU/l
Alanine aminotransferase	23 IU/l	5–35 IU/l
Screening test for glandular fever	negative	

QUESTION

- Suggest some possible diagnoses.

ANSWER 17

This seems likely to be an infective problem which has gone on for over a week. This makes influenza less likely. The other positive features are the lymphadenopathy and the oral ulceration. The temperature is still up and there has been a rash which has resolved. The blood results are all normal including the test for glandular fever (infectious mononucleosis) which was a reasonable diagnosis with these features.

The previous homosexual contact increases the possibility of sexually transmitted infections. He is known to have had a negative HIV test six months ago. However, it is quite possible that this might be an **HIV seroconversion illness**. In around half of those who acquire the virus this occurs within four to six weeks of acquisition. Although the HIV test will still be negative, this can be diagnosed by finding the presence of the HIV virus or its p24 antigen in the blood. He should have been counselled about precautions to reduce the risk of transmission of sexually transmitted diseases at the time of the HIV testing six months before.

The picture might fit for secondary syphilis which occurs six to eight weeks after the primary lesion. However, in that case the rash would often be more extensive and the lymph nodes are not usually tender. A serological test for syphilis should certainly be performed.

Other viral illnesses are possible. Hepatitis may present with this more general prodrome but the normal liver function tests make this much less likely.

In this case, tests for an HIV viraemia were positive. Antiretroviral treatment at the time of known or high-risk exposure is useful in reducing the risk of infection. At this stage, treatment is supportive with explanation and arrangements for monitoring of viral load.

KEY POINTS

- A seroconversion illness occurs in 50 per cent of those who acquire HIV infection. The severity varies.
- In cases of known or high-risk exposure, such as needlestick injuries, an immediate course of antiretroviral treatment is often indicated. Immediate advice should be sought.

A 60-year-old man presents with pain in the legs. The pain began six weeks ago and has been increasing in intensity. It is located around the ankles and is associated with local tenderness. He has been taking paracetamol for the pain in the legs but this has not been very effective and he wants to have some more effective pain killers.

There is no history of any joint problems in the past except for episodes of mild low back pain over the last 30 years. This has not been troubling him for five years or more. There is no other relevant previous medical history.

He smokes 20 cigarettes per day and drinks 15–20 units of alcohol each week. He works as a security guard and he is finding this difficult because of the pain in the legs. On routine questioning, he says that there has been no disturbance of bowels or micturition. His appetite has been less good over the last month; his weight is constant. There has been no chest pain. He has had a morning cough for many years. This has been more persistent throughout the day over the last eight weeks and he has produced small amounts of white sputum and, on one occasion, some streaks of blood in the sputum.

On examination, there is marked tenderness around the lower legs above the ankles and knees. There is slight tenderness around the wrists on both sides. There are crackles at the left base posteriorly in the chest. There is nothing else abnormal to find on examination except for clubbing of the fingers, although he says he has not noticed any change in the fingers.

A chest X-ray and X-rays of the knees are shown in Figs 18.1 to 18.3.

QUESTION

- What is the likely diagnosis?

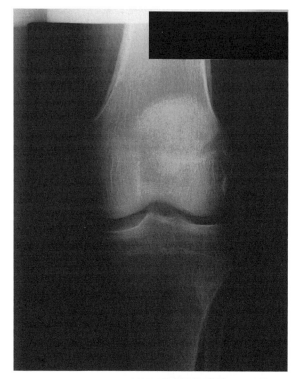

Figure 18.1
X-ray of knee joint

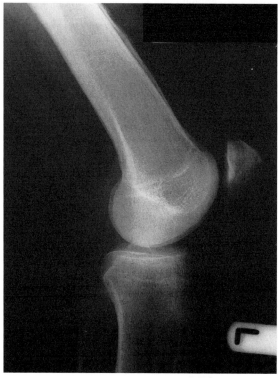

Figure 18.2
X-ray of knee joint

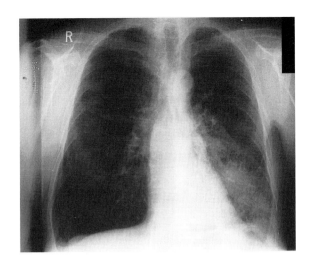

Figure 18.3 Chest X-ray

ANSWER 18

This case is likely to represent **carcinoma of the bronchus** associated with the non-metastatic manifestation of *hypertrophic pulmonary osteoarthropathy* (HPOA).

The chest X-ray shows consolidation in the left lower lobe with some loss of volume as shown by movement of the heart to the left. The chest X-ray could represent pneumonia but the story of the change in cough for eight weeks is rather long and the loss of volume on the X-ray is suspicious that there may be a lesion partly narrowing an airway. Consolidation classically is not associated with volume loss, because air in the alveoli is replaced by an inflammatory exudate. The single episode of haemoptysis in a 60-year-old smoker must always be regarded with a high degree of suspicion and investigated at least with a chest X-ray even though single episodes of streaks of blood in the sputum in the presence of a prominent cough are most often not associated with underlying malignancy. In this case the presence of finger clubbing adds to the suspicion. Patients often do not notice changes that come on slowly such as finger clubbing or say that the nails have always been the same.

On the X-rays around the knees, the appearance of elevation of the periostium around the outside borders of the femur is characteristic of HPOA. This painful condition is seen most often at the end of the long bones. Clubbing is usually present and it is nearly always associated with an underlying carcinoma of the lung, usually squamous cell or adenocarcinoma. The mechanism is not known and it can occasionally occur with other causes of clubbing such as intrathoracic sepsis. There is marked local tenderness with some local swelling. The pain is often difficult to control although it may resolve after thoracotomy even if complete resection at operation proves to be impossible.

In this case, bronchoscopy and biopsy showed adenocarcinoma of the lung and computed tomography (CT) scan showed that this was not resectable. Treatment with chemotherapy resulted in a temporary improvement in the chest X-ray but the leg pain continued to prove difficult to control.

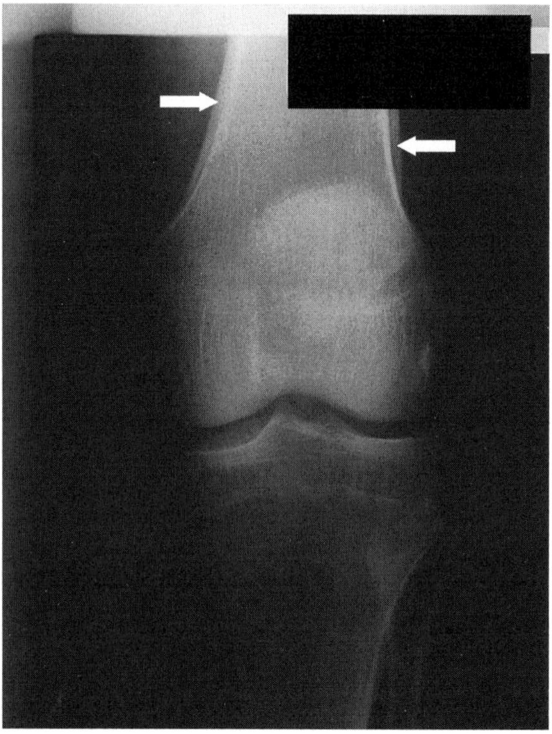

Figure 18.1 X-ray of knee joint (periosteal elevation arrowed)

- Change in the nature of a chronic cough in a smoker should be investigated.
- Carcinoma of the bronchus can present with non-metastatic manifestations related to endocrine, neurological and haematological abnormalities as well as clubbing and HPOA.

A 36-year-old woman presents to the casualty department with a 2-day history of left-sided loin pain associated with macroscopic haematuria. The pain is continuous and dull in character. Since her early twenties she has had previous episodes of loin pain which have occurred on both sides and resolved spontaneously over a few days. She has never passed any stones. She was noted to be mildly hypertensive during her two pregnancies. She has no other significant medical history. Her father died of a sub-arachnoid haemorrhage, aged 48. She has no siblings. Her two children, aged 12 and 10, are well. She works as a teacher and neither smokes or drinks alcohol.

On examination she is afebrile. Her pulse is regular at 84/min and her blood pressure is 145/100. Examination of the cardiovascular and respiratory systems is otherwise unremarkable. On palpation of her abdomen, a mass is palpable in each flank. These are not tender. Percussion is resonant over the areas and the masses are ballotable. Neurological examination is normal. Fundoscopy shows arteriovenous nipping and silver-wiring of the retinal vessels.

INVESTIGATIONS

		Normal
Haemoglobin	15.3 g/dl	(11.7–15.7 g/dl)
White cell count	6.2×10^9/l	($3.5–11.0 \times 10^9$/l)
Platelets	280×10^9/l	($150–440 \times 10^9$/l)
Sodium	136 mmol/l	(135–145 mmol/l)
Potassium	4.7 mmol/l	(3.5–5.0 mmol/l)
Urea	11.2 mmol/l	(2.5–6.7 mmol/l)
Creatinine	176 μmol/l	(70–120 μmol/l)
Albumin	45 g/l	(35–50g/l)

Urinalysis	+ protein; + + + blood
Urine microscopy	> 200 red cells; 10 white cells; no organisms
Abdominal X-ray	no intra-abdominal calcification seen

QUESTIONS

- What is the most likely diagnosis?
- How would you proceed to manage and investigate this patient?

ANSWER 19

The patient's history and examination is consistent with **autosomal dominant polycystic kidney disease** (ADPKD). She has macroscopic haematuria, hypertension and impaired renal function. The palpable abdominal masses in both flanks have the characteristic features of enlarged kidneys. In the left flank, an enlarged kidney may be confused with a large spleen although the latter will usually be dull to percussion and not ballotable. Other causes for palpable kidneys are renal cell carcinoma and massive hydronephrosis.

Although the name 'ADPKD' is derived from renal manifestations of cyst growth leading to enlarged kidneys and renal failure, it is a systemic disorder manifested by the presence of hepatic cysts, diverticular disease, inguinal hernias, mitral valve prolapse, intracranial aneurysms and hypertension. Flank pain is the most common symptom, and may be caused by cyst rupture, cyst infection or renal calculi. Macroscopic haematuria due to cyst haemorrhage occurs commonly and usually resolves spontaneously. Renal calculi occur in approximately 20 per cent of ADPKD patients (most commonly uric acid stones). Hypertension occurs early in the course of this disease affecting 60 per cent of patients with normal renal function. Approximately 50 per cent ADPKD patients will develop end-stage renal failure. Although it is not known if this patient's father had renal disease, it is highly likely that he had ADPKD and an associated berry aneurysm as the cause for his subarachnoid haemorrhage.

Ultrasonography is the preferred screening technique as it is cheap, non-invasive and rapid. It detects cysts as small as 0.5 cm. For a certain diagnosis, there should be at least three renal cysts with at least one cyst in each kidney. Ultrasound in this patient

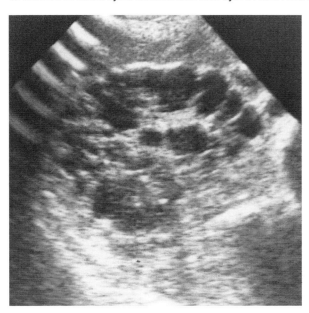

shows the typical appearance of multiple cysts (black areas) surrounded by thickened walls (Fig. 19.1). This patient should have blood and urine cultures performed to exclude an infected cyst. She should be referred to a nephrologist for long-term follow-up of her renal failure and plans made for renal replacement therapy. She needs to have effective blood pressure control with diastolic pressure < 85 mmHg to retard the progression of her renal failure. She should have MRI angiography to exclude an intracranial aneurysm. This

Figure 19.1 Renal ultrasound demonstrating multiple cysts

is not advocated for all ADPKD patients, but is indicated for those patients with a positive family history of aneurysm rupture. The patient's children should not be screened by ultrasound as at their age there is a high false-negative rate. By age 30, 90 per cent of ADPKD patients will have cysts detectable by ultrasound.

Ninety per cent of ADPKD patients have mutations in the ADPKD1 gene. This gene encodes for the protein polycystin which is a membrane glycoprotein which probably mediates cell–cell and/or cell–matrix interactions. Most remaining patients have mutations in the ADPKD2 gene which codes for polycystin-2, which has structural homology to polycystin and to calcium channels. ADPKD1 patients generally have an earlier age of onset of hypertension and development of renal failure as compared to ADPKD2 patients.

🔑 KEY POINTS

- ADPKD is the most common inherited renal disease, occurring in 1 : 600 to 1 : 1000 individuals.
- ADPKD patients may present with loin pain, haematuria, hypertension, renal failure or for counselling as asymptomatic relatives of affected individuals.

CASE 20

A 72-year-old lady is admitted to hospital because of increasing confusion. This has developed rapidly over the past three weeks and prior to this she had normal cognitive function. She also complains of loss of her appetite, headache and muscle cramps. She has long-standing hypertension and was started on bendrofluazide 5 mg once a day one month ago. She lives with her husband and neither drinks alcohol nor smokes. She is on no other medication.

On examination her skin turgor is normal. Her pulse is 80/min regular, blood pressure 160/100, jugular venous pressure normal, heart sounds normal with no peripheral oedema. Respiratory and abdominal systems are normal. She is disorientated in time, place and person. There is no focal neurology. Fundoscopy shows silver-wiring and arteriovenous nipping but no papilloedema.

INVESTIGATIONS

		Normal
Haemoglobin	12.2 g/dl	(11.7–15.7 g/dl)
White cell count	6.2×10^9/l	($3.5–11.0 \times 10^9$/l)
Platelets	172×10^9/l	($150–440 \times 10^9$/l)
Sodium	112 mmol/l	(135–145 mmol/l)
Potassium	3.2 mmol/l	(3.5–5.0 mmol/l)
Urea	3.2 mmol/l	(2.5–6.7 mmol/l)
Creatinine	64 μmol/l	(70–120 μmol/l)
Glucose	4.4 mmol/l	(4.0–6.0 mmol/l)
Albumin	37 g/l	(35–50g/l)
Urinary osmolality	320 mosmol/kg	(60–1200 mosmol/kg)
Urinary sodium	55 mmol/l	(5–300 mmol/l)
Urinalysis	no protein; no blood	
Chest X-ray	normal	

QUESTIONS

- What is the likely cause of this patient's confusion?
- How would you correct this problem?

ANSWER 20

This lady's confusion is due to **hyponatraemia**. There are many causes of confusion in the elderly but the very low sodium level in this case is an adequate explanation. Her serum is profoundly hypo-osmolar. In her case, it can be calculated from the following equation: $2 \times [Na+K] + urea + glucose = 238$ mosmol/kg (normal 278–305 mosmol/kg). Hyponatraemia may be asymptomatic but when it falls rapidly or reaches very low levels (below 120 mosmol/kg) can cause confusion, anorexia, cramps, fits and coma.

In most cases, hyponatraemia is due to excess retention of water. Normally, the dilutional fall in plasma osmolality suppresses antidiuretic hormone (ADH) secretion which allows excretion of excess water. In rare cases of primary polydipsia, the huge water intake may overwhelm this mechanism, and in severe renal failure the kidneys cannot excrete a water load but in most other cases of hyponatraemia there is an inability to suppress ADH secretion normally.

> **!** **CAUSES OF ELEVATED ADH**
>
> - Effective circulating volume depletion
>   True volume depletion – gastrointestinal, urinary and blood losses
>   Congestive cardiac failure and hepatic cirrhosis
>   Thiazide diuretics
> - Syndrome of inappropriate ADH secretion (SIADH)
> - Hormonal changes – Addison's disease, hypothyroidism, pregnancy

The low plasma sodium, potassium and urea in this patient are consistent with water excess. Measurement of urinary sodium and osmolality is useful. In primary polydipsia the urine can be maximally diluted to < 100 mosmol/kg, whereas in states with excess ADH the osmolality is usually > 320 mosmol/kg. Urinary sodium is usually < 25 mmol/l in hypovolaemic states, but > 40mmol/l in SIADH where patients are normovolaemic and the rate of sodium excretion depends on dietary intake and taking of diuretics. Diuretic-induced hyponatraemia tends to occur within a few weeks of starting treatment, and occurs mainly in elderly women often concurrently on non-steroidal anti-inflammatory drugs (NSAIDs) which inhibit water excretion. The clinical and biochemical picture in this woman is consistent with **diuretic-induced hyponatraemia**.

The rate of correction of hyponatraemia is controversial and must be tailored for individual patients. Hyponatraemia itself causes cell swelling, cerebral oedema, neurological dysfunction and damage. The brain counteracts this by exporting solutes (including potassium and organic osmolytes). Too rapid correction can induce neurological damage by causing central pontine myelinolysis. The MRI scan (Fig. 20.1) shows a high signal in the pons (arrow) consistent with pontine myelinolysis. The severity and duration of hyponatraemia as well as the presence of symptoms should be taken into account. Fluid restriction is sufficient in patients with a sodium > 120 mmol/l. Acutely hyponatraemic patients with a sodium < 120mmol/l should be corrected more rapidly than chronically hyponatraemic (< 120mmol/l), asymptomatic patients. This patient is chronically hyponatraemic (< 120mmol/l) with neurological

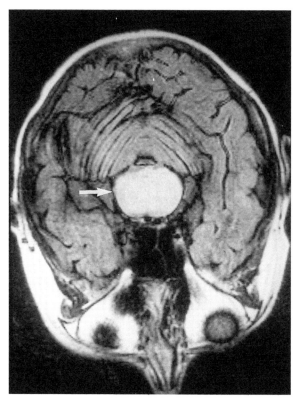

Figure 20.1 MRI scan of T1 weighted coronal image

symptoms. The diuretic should be stopped. The hyponatraemia should be corrected with isotonic saline at a maximum rate of rise of sodium of <0.5 mmol/h until the sodium has reached 130 mmol/l. Fluid restriction will then suffice to return the sodium slowly into the normal range.

⚷ KEY POINTS

- Hyponatraemia ia almost always due to water excess.
- Too rapid correction of hyponatraemia can cause neurological damage.
- There is very wide variation in urinary sodium excretion which depends in part on the dietary sodium intake.

CASE 21

A 46-year-old secretary presents to her GP complaining of headaches. These have become progressively more severe over the past three months. The headaches are frontal, worse in the morning and exacerbated by coughing. She has also noticed that her vision in both eyes has deteriorated recently. She has had some pain in the hands and forearms at night. She has become aware that it is difficult to remove her wedding ring from her finger, and that she needs a larger size in gloves and shoes. She feels that her facial appearance has changed over the past few years with coarsening of her features. She has no significant past medical history. She is married, smokes 20 cigarettes a day and drinks an average of 12 units of alcohol per week. She takes paracetamol regularly for her headaches.

On examination, she has coarse facial features and large hands. Her pulse is 84/min regular, blood pressure 160/100. Examination of her cardiovascular, respiratory and abdominal systems is otherwise normal. Visual field examination reveals some loss of the temporal field in each eye. Fundoscopy demonstrates optic atrophy.

INVESTIGATIONS

		Normal
Haemoglobin	12.2 g/dl	(11.7–15.7 g/dl)
Mean cell volume	86 fl	(80–99 fl)
White cell count	6.7×10^9/l	($3.5–11.0 \times 10^9$/l)
Platelets	248×10^9/l	($150–440 \times 10^9$/l)
Sodium	137 mmol/l	(135–145 mmol/l)
Potassium	3.8 mmol/l	(3.5–5.0 mmol/l)
Bicarbonate	27 mmol/l	(24–30 mmol/l)
Urea	5.2 mmol/l	(2.5–6.7 mmol/l)
Creatinine	98 μmol/l	(70–120 μmol/l)
Glucose	8.2 mmol/l	(4.0–6.0 mmol/l)
Urinalysis	no blood; no protein; +++ glucose	

QUESTIONS

- What is the diagnosis?
- How would you investigate and manage this patient?

ANSWER 21

The clinical features suggest that this woman has **acromegaly** due to a growth hormone-secreting pituitary tumour. The change in facial appearance, symptoms suggesting carpal tunnel syndrome, visual signs, hypertension and hyperglycaemia are characteristic. About one-third of patients with acromegaly may present because they notice a change in their facial appearance, another one-third have associated disturbances such as visual field defects, carpal tunnel syndrome or headaches, and the remainder are recognized to be acromegalic when seeking medical attention for another reason. Carbohydrate metabolism is often disturbed leading to hyperglycaemia and glycosuria. This is because growth hormone antagonizes the insulin-mediated cell uptake of glucose.

Other causes for enlarged hands include regular manual work, obesity, hypothyroidism and amyloidosis. Visual field defects are an important early symptom of a pituitary tumour. Bitemporal hemianopia due to optic chiasm compression may be caused by upward extension of pituitary tumours, or by craniopharyngiomas and suprasellar meningiomas. Central chiasmatic lesions produce symmetrical bitemporal field loss and progress to optic atrophy with reduced central visual acuity. Papilloedema is rare unless extension into the third ventricle has caused hydrocephalus.

The patient should be referred to an endocrinologist for investigation. A helpful clue to the diagnosis is to obtain photographs of the patient at an earlier age to see if her features have really changed over the course of the time. The diagnosis is confirmed by finding a raised growth hormone (GH) level that does not suppress normally in a glucose suppression test. The following hormones should be assayed to exclude deficiency caused by compression by the GH-secreting adenoma: luteinizing hormone/follicle-stimulating hormone (LH/FSH), oestradiol (in females), testosterone (in males), thyroxine and thyroid-stimulating hormone (TSH), prolactin and cortisol. A combined pituitary stimulation test may be needed. A MRI scan (T1-weighted coronal image) through the pituitary following intravenous contrast medium (gadolinium-DTPA) (Fig. 21.1) shows a macroadenoma replacing the normal gland (long arrow) and showing rim enhancement (short arrow).

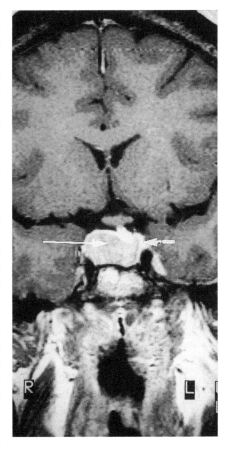

Figure 21.1 MRI scan of T1 weighted coronal image

Various treatments are available including surgery (transsphenoidal hypophysectomy or adenoma removal), external radiotherapy or yttrium-90 implantation. Bromocriptine lowers GH levels but is generally reserved for patients unfit for surgery since symptoms related to pressure from the tumour are unaffected. The patient needs long-term endocrine follow-up because of the risk of hypopituitarism.

> **🔍 KEY POINTS**
>
> - Acromegaly may present with altered appearance, headaches or visual loss.
> - Coarse facial features may be normal and old photographs help to confirm a change in appearance.
> - The diagnosis of acromegaly is confirmed by finding a raised growth hormone level (GH) that does not suppress normally in a glucose suppression test.

CASE 22

A 43-year-old woman presents to her GP complaining of pains in her joints. She has noticed these pains worsening over several months. Her joints are most stiff on waking in the mornings. The joints that are most painful are the small joints of the hands and feet. The pain is relieved by diclofenac tablets. She is otherwise well and has had no serious medical illnesses. She is married with two children and works as a legal secretary. She is a non-smoker and drinks alcohol only occasionally. Her only medication is diclofenac.

On examination she looks well. Her proximal interphalangeal joints and metacarpophalangeal joints are swollen and painful with effusions present. Her metatarsophalangeal joints are also tender. Physical examination is otherwise normal.

INVESTIGATIONS

		Normal
Haemoglobin	8.4 g/dl	(11.7–15.7 g/dl)
Mean cell volume	87 fl	(80.5–99.7 fl)
White cell count	7.2×10^9/l	($3.5–11.0 \times 10^9$/l)
Platelets	438×10^9/l	($150–440 \times 10^9$/l)
Erythrocyte sedimentation rate	46 mm/h	(<10 mm/h)
Sodium	143 mmol/l	(135–145 mmol/l)
Potassium	3.7 mmol/l	(3.5–5.0 mmol/l)
Urea	5.7 mmol/l	(2.5–6.7 mmol/l)
Creatinine	84 μmol/l	(70–120 μmol/l)
Glucose	4.6 mmol/l	(4.0–6.0 mmol/l)
Albumin	39 g/l	(35–50 g/l)
Urinalysis	no protein; no blood; no glucose	

QUESTIONS

- What is the diagnosis and the major differential diagnoses?
- How would you investigate and manage this patient?

ANSWER 22

This patient has symptoms and signs typical of early **rheumatoid arthritis**. Rheumatoid arthritis is a chronic, systemic inflammatory disorder principally affecting joints in a peripheral symmetrical distribution. Rheumatoid arthritis characteristically affects proximal interphalangeal, metacarpophalangeal and wrist joints in the hands. It is a disease with a long course with exacerbations and remissions. It may present acutely as part of a systemic illness or more chronically with joint stiffness. Extra-articular features include rheumatoid nodules, vasculitis causing cutaneous nodules and digital gangrene, scleritis, pleural effusions, diffuse pulmonary fibrosis, pulmonary nodules, obliterative bronchiolitis, pericarditis and splenomegaly (Felty's syndrome). There is usually a normochromic normocytic anaemia and raised erythrocyte sedimentation rate (ESR) as seen here.

❗ DIFFERENTIAL DIAGNOSIS OF AN ACUTE SYMMETRICAL POLYARTHRITIS

- Osteoarthritis (characteristically affects distal interphalangeal as well as proximal interphalangeal and first metacarpophalangeal joints).
- Systemic lupus erythematosus (usually causes a mild, flitting non-erosive arthritis).
- Gout (usually starts as a monoarthritis).
- Seronegative arthritides (ankylosing spondylitis, psoriasis, Reiter's disease). These usually cause an asymmetrical arthritis affecting medium and larger joints as well as sacroiliac and distal interphalangeal joints).
- Acute viral arthritis (e.g rubella – resolves completely).

This patient should be referred to a rheumatologist for further investigation and management. The affected joints should be X-rayed (Fig. 22.1). If there has been joint damage, the X-rays will show subluxation, juxta-articular osteoporosis, loss of joint space and bony erosions. A common site for erosions to be found in early rheumatoid arthritis is the fifth metatarsophalangeal joint (arrow). Blood tests should be taken for rheumatoid factor (present in rheumatoid arthritis) and anti-DNA antibodies (present in systemic lupus erythematosus). The patient should be given non-steroidal anti-inflammatory drugs for analgesia and to reduce joint stiffness to allow her to continue her secretarial work. Disease-modifying drugs such as gold or penicillamine should be considered unless the patient settles easily on non-steroidal anti-inflammatory drugs.

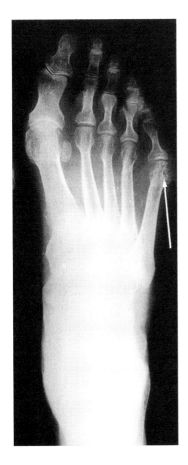

Figure 22.1 X-ray of foot

- Rheumatoid arthritis does not typically affect distal interphalangeal joints.
- Systemic symptoms of rheumatoid arthritis may precede the joint symptoms.

A 38-year-old woman presents to the casualty department with an acutely swollen left leg. She had woken that morning to notice that her leg was painful and swollen to the level of the thigh. There was no history of recent air travel or long distance car journeys. She is otherwise well and is not breathless and has no chest pain. She has had no previous medical illnesses but in her obstetric history she has had five first trimester miscarriages and has not had any successful pregnancies. There is no family history of note. The patient is married. She is a teacher and neither smokes tobacco nor drinks alcohol. The oral contraceptive is the only medication that she takes.

On examination, she is overweight. Her left leg is clearly swollen, with a 9-cm difference in circumference around the upper thigh. There is tenderness on palpation of her left calf muscles. The left leg is warmer with engorged superficial veins. Physical examination is otherwise normal.

INVESTIGATIONS

		Normal
Haemoglobin	12.2 g/dl	(11.7–15.7 g/dl)
Mean cell volume	86 fl	(80–99 fl)
White cell count	7.4×10^9/l	($3.5–11.0 \times 10^9$/l)
Platelets	328×10^9/l	($150–440 \times 10^9$/l)
Sodium	141 mmol/l	(135–145 mmol/l)
Potassium	4.6 mmol/l	(3.5–5.0 mmol/l)
Urea	4.9 mmol/l	(2.5–6.7 mmol/l)
Creatinine	111 μmol/l	(70–120 μmol/l)
Glucose	4.8 mmol/l	(4.0–6.0 mmol/l)
Prothrombin time		normal
Activated partial thromboplastin time		prolonged

QUESTIONS

- What is the cause of the swollen leg?
- How would you investigate and manage this patient?

ANSWER 23

This patient has a clinical diagnosis of a left **deep-vein thrombosis** (DVT). The main differential diagnoses of an acutely swollen leg are a ruptured Baker's cyst and acute cellulitis. Other causes of chronically swollen legs are obesity, lymphoedema, congestive cardiac failure and previous DVTs (postphlebitic).

! MAJOR RISK FACTORS FOR DVTs

- Dehydration, prolonged inactivity, bedrest, post-surgical, obesity.
- Malignancy – cancers of the lung, pancreas, breast, prostate and gut are particularly associated. Pelvic malignancy causing compression can directly lead to venous thrombosis.
- Oral contraceptives – oestrogens increase the risk.
- Genetic causes – protein C/S deficiency, antithrombin III deficiency, homocystinuria and factor V Leiden mutation.
- Behçet's syndrome – a diagnostic triad of iritis, orogenital ulceration and DVTs.
- Antiphospholipid antibody syndrome.

When a patient presenting with a DVT is young, or where there is no obvious underlying cause or where there is a strong family history or a history of recurrent events underlying risk factors should be investigated. This woman had obesity, oral contraceptive use and the presence of antiphospholipid antibodies as risk factors for her DVT. Antiphospholipid antibodies may be present as part of systemic lupus erythematosus (SLE) or may be an isolated finding, primary antiphospholipid antibody syndrome. Although the antibodies prolong the activated partial thromboplastin time (APTT) they predispose to thrombosis. Recurrent miscarriages, as in this patient, may be a feature. Patients may present with idiopathic recurrent DVT, arterial gangrene, livedo reticularis, cerebral infarcts, chorea and multi-infarct dementia.

Doppler ultrasound of her femoral veins will confirm the diagnosis of DVT. Her pelvis should also be scanned to exclude a mass. A thrombophilia screen should be sent. Lupus serology should also be performed to define if the antiphospholipid antibodies are part of SLE in this patient.

This patient should be immediately anticoagulated either with intravenous heparin or subcutaneous low-molecular-weight heparin to prevent proximal propagation of the thrombus and pulmonary emboli. The patient should be started on warfarin. Patients with antiphospholipid antibodies require life-long anticoagulation to prevent further thrombotic events.

⚲ KEY POINTS

- Young patients with venous thromboses should be investigated for underlying causes.
- Patients with antiphospholipid antibodies require life-long anticoagulation.

A 44-year-old woman presents to her GP complaining of headaches. These headaches have been present in previous years but have now become more intense. She describes the headaches as severe and present on both sides of her head. They tend to worsen during the course of the day. There is no associated visual disturbance or vomiting. She also complains of loss of appetite and difficulty sleeping with early morning waking. She has had eczema and irritable bowel syndrome diagnosed in the past but these are not giving her problems at the moment. She is divorced with two children aged 10 and 12 whom she looks after. She has a part-time job as an office cleaner. Her mother has recently died of a brain tumour. She smokes about 20 cigarettes per day and drinks 15 units of alcohol per week. She takes regular paracetamol or ibuprofen for her headaches.

On examination she looks withdrawn. Her pulse is 74/min and regular, blood pressure is 118/76. Examinations of cardiovascular, respiratory and gastrointestinal systems, breasts and reticuloendothelial system are normal. There are no abnormal neurological signs and fundoscopy is normal.

QUESTIONS

- What is the diagnosis?
- What are the major differential diagnoses?
- How would you manage this patient?

ANSWER 24

This patient has a **chronic tension headache**. This is the commonest form of headache. It occurs mainly in patients under the age of 50 years. The headache is usually bilateral often with diffuse radiation over the vertex of the skull, although it may be more localized. The pain is often characterized as a sense of pressure on the head. Visual symptoms and vomiting do not occur. The pain is often at its worst in the evening. Patients may show symptoms of depression (this woman has biological symptoms of loss of appetite and disturbed sleep pattern). Sufferers may reveal sources of stress such as bereavement or difficulty with work. There may be an element of suggestion as in this case, with concern that she may have inherited a brain tumour from her mother. She is looking after two children alone and working part time. A normal neurological examination is important for reassurance.

! MAJOR ALTERNATIVE DIAGNOSIS OF CHRONIC HEADACHES

- Classic migraine – characterized by visual symptoms followed within 30 min by the onset of severe hemicranial throbbing, headache, photophobia, nausea and vomiting lasting for several hours. The onset is usually in early adult life and a positive family history may be present.
- Cluster headaches – mainly affect men. The pain is unilateral, usually orbital and severe in nature. It characteristically occurs 1–2 hours after sleeping, and lasts 1–2 hours and recurs nightly for six to eight weeks.
- Headache caused by a space-occupying lesion (such as tumour or abscess). Often the headache is initially mild but over a few weeks becomes severe and is exacerbated by coughing or sneezing. The headache is usually worse in the morning and is associated with vomiting. There will often be other signs, including personality change and focal neurological signs.
- Miscellaneous causes – sinusitis, dental disorders, cervical spondylosis, glaucoma, post-traumatic headache.

It is important to come to a clear diagnosis and to address the patient's beliefs and concerns about the symptoms. In some circumstances it may be necessary to perform a computed tomography (CT) head scan for reassurance. The question of depression needs to be explored further and may need treating with antidepressants.

⚷ KEY POINTS

- Tension headaches occur mainly in the under fifties and patients often show features of depression.

CASE 25

A 32-year-old woman is complaining of chest pain. This had been present for two years on and off. The pain settled for a period of six months but it has returned over the last ten months. The pain is usually on the left side of the chest, radiating to the left axilla. She describes it as a tight or gripping pain which lasts for anything from 5 to 30 min at a time. It can come on at any time, often related to exercise but it has occurred at rest on some occasions, particularly in the evenings. The pain is usually associated with shortness of breath. It makes her stop whatever she is doing and she often feels faint or dizzy with the pain. Occasionally palpitations come on after the start of the pain. Detailed questioning about the palpitations indicates that they are a sensation of a strong but steady heart beat.

In her previous medical history she had her appendix removed at the age of 15 years. At the age of 30 years she was investigated for an irregular bowel habit and abdominal pain but no specific diagnosis was arrived at. These symptoms still trouble her. She has seasonal rhinitis. Two years ago she visited a chemist and had her cholesterol level measured; the result was 4.3 mmol/l (desired level < 5.5 mmol/l). In her family history her grandfather died of a myocardial infarction, a year previously, aged 77. Several members of her family had hayfever or asthma. She works as a medical secretary. She is married and has no children.

On examination, she has a blood pressure of 112/68, pulse of 78/min which is regular. The heart sounds are normal. There is some tenderness on the left side of the chest, to the left of the sternum and in the left submammary area. The respiratory rate is 22/min. No abnormalities were found on examination of the lungs. She is tender in the left iliac fossa.

Her ECG is shown (Fig. 25.1).

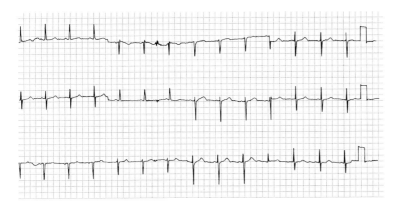

Figure 25.1

She asked to be referred for a coronary arteriogram to rule out significant coronary artery disease.

QUESTION

- What should be done?

ANSWER 25

The ECG shown is normal. **The pain does not have the characteristics of ischaemic heart disease**. On the basis of the information given here it would be reasonable to explore her anxieties and to reassure the patient that this is very unlikely to represent coronary artery disease and to assess subsequently the effects of that reassurance. It may well be that she is anxious about the death of her grandfather from ischaemic heart disease. He may have had symptoms before his death which were related to her anxieties. From a risk point of view her grandfather's death at the age of 77 with no other affected relatives is not a relevant risk factor. She has expressed anxiety already by having the cholesterol measured (and found to be normal).

She has a history which is suspicious of irritable bowel syndrome with persistent pain and irregular bowel habit and normal investigations. Ischaemic chest pain is usually central and generally reproducible with the same stimuli. The associated shortness of breath may reflect overventilation coming on with the pain and giving her dizziness and palpitations.

The characteristics of the pain and associated shortness of breath should be explored further. Asthma can sometimes be described as tightness or pain in the chest and she has seasonal rhinitis and a family history of asthma.

Gastrointestinal causes of pain such as reflux oesophagitis are unlikely in view of the site and relation on occasions to exercise. The length of the history excludes other causes of acute chest pain such as pericarditis.

The problem of embarking on tests is that there is no simple screening test which can rule out significant coronary artery disease. Too many investigations may reinforce her belief in her illness and false-positive findings do occur and may exacerbate her anxieties. However, if the patient could not be simply reassured it might be appropriate to proceed with an exercise stress test or a thallium scan to look for areas of reversible ischaemia on exercise or other stress. A coronary arteriogram would not be appropriate without other information to indicate a higher degree of risk of coronary artery disease.

KEY POINTS

- Ischaemic heart disease characteristically causes central rather than left-sided chest pain.
- The resting ECG may show signs of ischaemia or previous infarction but is not a very sensitive test for ischaemic heart disease.

A 40-year-old man has a two-month history of abdominal pain. The pain is epigastric or central and is intermittent. He had a similar episode a year before. On that occasion he took some indigestion mixture obtained from a retail pharmacy and the symptoms resolved after ten weeks. The pain usually lasts for 30 to 60 min. It often occurs at night, when it can wake him up, and seems to improve after meals. Some foods such as curries and other spicey foods seem to bring on the pain on occasions.

He had smoked 15 cigarettes per day for 25 years and drinks around 24 units of alcohol each week. He is not taking any medication at present. There is no other relevant medical history. He works as a financial broker in the City. He has been feeling more tired recently and had put this down to pressure of work. A blood count was sent.

BLOOD TESTS

		Normal
Haemoglobin	10.1 g/dl	13.3–17.7 g/dl
Red cell count	$6.4 \times 10^{12}/l$	$4.4–5.9 \times 10^{12}/l$
Mean corpuscular volume (MCV)	72 fl	80.5–99.7 fl
White cell count	$9.8 \times 10^9/l$	$3.9–10.6 \times 10^9/l$
Platelet count	$300 \times 10^9/l$	$150–440 \times 10^9/l$
Iron	4 μmol/l	14–31 μmol/l
Total iron-binding capacity	76 μmol/l	45–70 μmol/l
Ferritin	7μg/l	20–300 μg/l

The blood film is reported as showing microcytic, hypochromic red cells.

QUESTIONS

- How do you interpret these findings?
- What is the likely diagnosis and how should it be confirmed?

ANSWER 26

The blood count shows anaemia with a low mean corpuscular volume (MCV) indicating a microcytic anaemia. The high red cell count with low haemoglobin shows that the haemoglobin content of the cells is reduced. The low serum iron and ferritin with a high total iron-binding capacity (TIBC) confirm that this is related to true iron deficiency. The blood film confirms that the cells are microcytic and low in haemoglobin (hypochromasia). In anaemia of chronic disease the cells may be microcytic and serum iron low but the TIBC would be low also and ferritin normal. The diagnosis is most likely to be a **peptic ulcer**.

The commonest cause of iron-deficiency anaemia in a man is gastrointestinal blood loss. In a premenopausal woman menstrual blood loss would be the most common cause. The abdominal pains would be consistent with those from a peptic ulcer, especially a duodenal ulcer when there is more often some relief from food. The diagnosis should be established by endoscopy because alternative diagnoses such as carcinoma of the stomach cannot be ruled out from the history. The site of the blood loss causing the iron deficiency should be established. At the same time the presence of *Helicobacter pylori* should be investigated.

In this case, an endoscopy confirmed an active duodenal ulcer and samples were positive for *Helicobacter pylori*. This is associated with gastritis and peptic ulceration. Tests of expired breath and serum antibodies are alternative diagnostic tests. The *H. pylori* was treated by a combined regime of omeprazole for six weeks and triple therapy with De-Nol, amoxycillin and metronidazole for two weeks. He was given careful instructions not to drink while on the metronidazole since it has an antabuse-like action. He was given strong recommendations to stop smoking. The iron deficiency was corrected by additional oral iron which was continued for three months to replenish the iron stores in the bone marrow. Repeat endoscopy to show healing confirms the original diagnosis of benign ulceration.

⚲ KEY POINTS

- Various antibiotic regimes have been shown to temporarily remove *Helicobacter pylori* and prevent or postpone recurrence of symptoms and ulceration.
- Replenishment of iron stores in the bone marrow needs three months' treatment with oral iron after the haemoglobin has returned to normal.
- Ferritin is an acute-phase protein and will be raised in the presence of acute illness even in the presence of iron deficiency.

CASE 27

A 55-year-old man is admitted to hospital with headache and confusion. He has a cough and a temperature of 38.2°C. He did not complain of any other symptoms. On examination he looked thin and unwell and he was slightly drowsy. His mini mental test score was 8/10. There were some crackles in the upper zones of the chest posteriorly. His respiratory rate was 20/min. There were no neurological signs.

Two months earlier he had been admitted with a productive cough and acid-fast bacilli had been found in the sputum on direct smear. He had lost weight and complained of occasional night sweats. He had a history of a head injury ten years previously. He smoked 15 cigarettes a day and drank 40–60 units of alcohol each week. He was found a place in a local hostel for the homeless and sent out after one week in hospital on antituberculous treatment with rifampicin, isoniazid and pyrazinamide together with pyridoxine. His chest X-ray at the time showed patchy infiltration in the right upper lobe.

His chest X-ray is shown in Fig. 27.1.

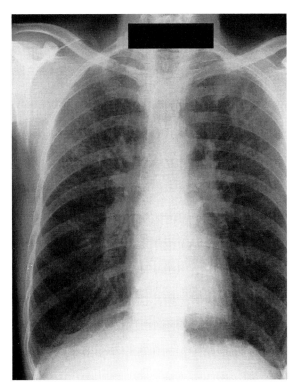

Figure 27.1

QUESTION

• What might be the cause of his second admission?

ANSWER 27

The chest X-ray shows extensive changes in the upper zones which seem as if they are likely to be more extensive than those described at the first admission two months earlier. It is likely that this is a worsening of his **pulmonary tuberculosis**. This might occur because he had a resistant organism or, more likely, because he had not taken his treatment as prescribed. Risk factors for development of tuberculosis are poor nutrition, high alcohol intake, immunosuppression (HIV, immunosuppressive therapy). Higher rates occur in those from the Indian subcontinent and parts of Africa.

The headache and confusion raise the possibility of tuberculous meningitis. Other possibilities would be liver damage from the antituberculous drugs and the alcohol, although clinical jaundice would be expected, or electrolyte imbalance. If these are not present a lumbar puncture would be indicated provided that there is no sign to suggest raised intracranial pressure. It would be advisable to do a computed tomography (CT) scan of the brain first since a fall related to his high alcohol consumption might have led to a subdural haemorrhage to give him his headache and confusion.

It is now two months since the initial finding of acid-fast bacilli in the sputum and the cultures and sensitivities of the organism should now be available. These should be checked to be sure that the organism was *Mycobacterium tuberculosis* and that it was sensitive to the three anti-tuberculous drugs which he was given. As a check on compliance, blood levels of anti-tuberculous drugs can be measured. The urine will be coloured orangy-red by metabolites of rifampicin taken in the last 8 hours or so.

Comparison with his old chest X-rays showed extension of the upper-lobe shadowing which is now bilateral. It is difficult to be sure about activity from a chest X-ray but extension of shadowing is obviously suspicious. 'Softer' more fluffy shadowing is more likely to be associated with active disease. A direct smear of the sputum showed that acid-fast bacilli were still present on direct smear. He confirmed that he was not taking his medication regularly. His headache and confusion resolved as he stopped his high alcohol intake. Subsequently the antituberculous therapy should be given as directly observed therapy (DOT) in a thrice-weekly regime supervised at each administration by a district nurse or health visitor.

⚒ KEY POINTS

- Poor adherence to treatment regimes is the commonest cause of failure of antituberculous and other treatment.
- Directly observed therapy should be used when there is any doubt about adherence to treatment.
- Four drugs should be used (rifampicin, isoniazid, pyrazinamide and ethambutol) when there is a higher risk of resistant organisms, e.g. immigrants from Africa, Asia, previously treated patients, patients of no fixed abode.

A 30-year-old woman is brought up to the accident & emergency department at 2 pm by her husband. He is worried that she has taken some tablets in an attempt to harm herself. She has a history suggestive of depression since the birth of her son three months earlier. She has been having some counselling since that time but has not been on any medication. The previous evening about 10 pm she told her husband that she was going to take some pills and locked herself in the bathroom. Two hours later he persuaded her to come out and she said that she had not taken anything. They went to bed but he has brought her up now because she has complained of a little nausea and he is worried that she might have taken something when she was in the bathroom.

The only tablets which he knows were in the house were aspirin, paracetamol and temazepam which he took occasionally for insomnia.

She complains of a little nausea although she has not vomited. She has had a little abdominal discomfort. There is no relevant previous medical or family history of note. She worked as a primary school teacher until 30 weeks of the pregnancy.

On examination she is mentally alert. She says that she feels sad. The pulse is 76/min, blood pressure is 124/78 and respiratory rate is 16/min. There is some mild abdominal tenderness in the upper abdomen but nothing else abnormal to find.

INVESTIGATIONS

		Normal
Haemoglobin	12.7 g/dl	11.7–15.7 g/dl
Mean corpuscular volume (MCV)	87 fl	80.8–100 fl
White cell count	6.8×10^9/l	$3.5–11.0 \times 10^9$/l
Platelet count	230×10^9/l	$150–440 \times 10^9$/l
International Normalized Ratio (INR) prothrombin time	18 s	10–14s
Sodium	139 mmol/l	135–145 mmol/l
Potassium	3.8 mmol/l	3.5–5.0 mmol/l
Urea	4.6 mmol/l	2.5–6.7 mmol/l
Creatinine	81 μmol/l	70–120 μmol/l
Alkaline phosphatase	88 IU/l	30–300 IU/l
Alanine aminotransferase (AAT)	37 IU/l	5–35 IU/l
Gamma-glutamyl transpeptidase	32 IU/l	11–51 IU/l
Glucose	5.1 mmol/l	4.0–6.0 mmol/l

QUESTION

- What should the management be now?

ANSWER 28

It is not evident from the history that the patient herself has been asked about any tablets or other agents she has taken. This would be an important area to be sure of. Of the three agents mentioned, the only one likely to be relevant is **paracetamol**. Aspirin and temazepam would be likely to produce more symptoms in less than 14 hours if they have been taken in significant quantity. However, the salicylate level should certainly be measured; in this case it was not raised. In the absence of drowsiness at this time, it is not necessary to consider temazepam any further.

The only significant abnormality on the blood tests is the slightly high International Normalized Ratio (INR) and minimally raised alanine aminotransferase (AAT). The INR increase is a signal that a paracetamol overdose is likely. It is often the first test to become abnormal when there is liver damage from paracetamol overdose. If the INR is normal at 24 hours then a significant problem is very likely. There are few symptoms in the first 24 hours except perhaps nausea, vomiting and abdominal discomfort. This may be associated with tenderness over the liver. The liver-function tests usually become abnormal after the first 24 hours.

The paracetamol level should be measured urgently; it was found to be high. The evidence of early liver damage from the INR would in itself suggest that treatment with acetylcysteine would be appropriate. The earlier this is used the better but it is certainly still worthwhile 16 hours after the ingestion. In this case a level of paracetamol of 64 mg/l confirmed that treatment was appropriate and that the risk of severe liver damage was high. Further advice can always be obtained by ringing one of the national Poisons Information Services. The electrolyte, renal and liver-function tests and the clotting studies should be monitored carefully over the first few days and referral to a liver unit considered if there is marked liver dysfunction.

The other areas which need to be addressed in this case are the mental state and the safety and care of the son and any other children. This is a *serious drug overdose*. She should be seen by a psychiatrist or other appropriately trained health worker. The question of any possible risk to the baby should be evaluated before she returns home.

ꭓ KEY POINTS

- Intravenous acetylcysteine and oral methionine are effective treatments for paracetamol overdose if started early enough.
- Paracetamol levels can be used to predict problems and guide treatment if the time since overdose is known.

CASE 29

A 23-year-old man presented with malaise and anorexia for one week. He has felt feverish but has not taken his temperature. For two weeks he has had aching pains in the knees, elbows and wrists without any obvious swelling of the joints.

Five years ago he had glandular fever confirmed serologically. He smokes 25 cigarettes per day and drinks 20–40 units of alcohol per week. He has taken marijuana and ecstasy occasionally over the past two years and various tablets and mixtures at clubs without being sure of the constituents. He denies any intravenous drug use. He has had protected homosexual contacts but says that he had an HIV test which was negative six months earlier.

He is unemployed and lives in a flat with three other people. There is no relevant family history.

On examination he has a temperature of 38.6°C and looks unwell. He looks as if he may be a little jaundiced. He is tender in the right upper quadrant of the abdomen. There are no abnormalities to find on examination of the joints or in any other system.

INVESTIGATIONS

		Normal
Haemoglobin	13.9 g/dl	13.3–17.7 g/dl
Mean corpuscular volume (MCV)	85 fl	80.5–99.7 fl
White cell count	11.3 × 10⁹/l	3.9–10.6 × 10⁹/l
Platelet count	286 × 10⁹/l	150–440 × 10⁹/l
Prothrombin time	18s	10–14s
Sodium	136 mmol/l	135–145 mmol/l
Potassium	3.5 mmol/l	3.5–5.0 mmol/l
Urea	3.2 mmol/l	2.5–6.7 mmol/l
Creatinine	65μmol/l	70–120 μmol/l
Bilirubin	55 μmol/l	3–17 μmol/l
Alkaline phosphatase	378 IU/l	30–300 IU/l
Alanine aminotransferase	560 IU/l	5–35 IU/l
Fasting glucose	4.2 mmol/l	4.0–6.0 mmol/l

QUESTIONS

- What is your interpretation of the findings?
- What is the likely diagnosis?
- What treatment is required?

ANSWER 29

The diagnosis is likely to be **acute viral hepatitis**. The biochemical results show abnormal liver-function tests with a predominant change in the transaminases. This might be caused by hepatitis A, B or C. The raised white count is compatible with acute hepatitis. Homosexuality and intravenous drug abuse are risk factors for hepatitis B and C. Other viral infections such as cytomegalovirus and herpes simplex virus are possible.

Since the drug ingestion history is unclear, there is a possibility of a drug-induced hepatitis. The prodromal joint symptoms suggest a viral infection as the cause and this is more common with hepatitis B. Serological tests can be used to see whether there are IgM antibodies indicating acute infection with one of these viruses to confirm the diagnosis. The reported negative HIV test six months earlier makes an HIV-associated condition unlikely although patients are not always reliable in their accounts of HIV tests.

Treatment is basically supportive in the acute phase. The prothrombin time in this patient is raised slightly but not enough to be an anxiety or an indicator of very severe disease. Liver function will need to be measured to monitor enzyme levels as a guide to progress. Alcohol and any other hepatotoxic drug intake should be avoided until liver-function tests are back to normal. If hepatitis B or C is confirmed by serology then liver-function tests and serological tests should be monitored for chronic disease and antiviral therapy then considered. Rare complications of the acute illness are fulminant hepatic failure, aplastic anaemia, myocarditis and vasculitis. The opportunity should be taken to advise him about the potential dangers of his intake of cigarettes, drugs and alcohol and to offer him appropriate support in these areas.

✎ KEY POINTS

- Viral hepatitis is often associated with a prodrome of arthralgia and flu-like symptoms.
- Confirmatory evidence should be sought for patients' reports of HIV test results.

CASE 30

A 53-year-old woman has recently noticed a black lesion on her right shin. The lesion is raised and about 1.5 cm in diameter. It seems to have enlarged rapidly in size over the past few weeks. The lesion bleeds if she scratches it. She otherwise feels well. She is married and has two children. She previously has lived in Australia for 20 years.

On examination she is Caucasian. There is a 1.5 × 1cm lesion on the anterior surface of her right lower leg. The lesion is black and raised with an irregular edge. There are two smaller lesions adjacent to it. There are two firm inguinal nodes palpable in her right groin. Physical examination is otherwise normal.

QUESTIONS

- What is the diagnosis?
- How would you investigate and manage this patient?

ANSWER 30

This woman has a **malignant melanoma** on her leg. Malignant melanoma is an invasive neoplastic disorder of melanocytes.

> **❗ DIFFERENTIAL DIAGNOSES OF LOCALIZED PIGMENTED SKIN LESIONS**
>
> - Solar keratoses (tend to be scaly and brown)
> - Seborrhoeic wart
> - Pigmented basal cell carcinoma
> - Pyogenic granuloma (tend to be redder and smaller than melanoma)
> - Melanocytic naevus (more uniform pigmentation than melanoma)
> - Vascular malformation

Melanomas are related to sun exposure and occur typically in sun-exposed parts of the body. They usually occur in Caucasians. This patient's time in Australia would increase her sun exposure and her risk of malignant melanoma. About 50 per cent of melanomas develop from a pre-existing melanocytic naevus and the rest develop *de novo*. The presence of uneven pigmentation, an irregular edge and satellite lesions is characteristic of melanoma. There is often erosion of the skin surface and bleeding. The lesion may be itchy. Lymphadenopathy implies lymphatic spread of the tumour. Melanomas are extremely malignant and metastasize rapidly. However, early lesions are easy to cure and it is vitally important that they are recognized and treated appropriately.

The most important determinant of prognosis is the depth of invasion into the dermis. When the lesion spreads horizontally it tends to be noted and treated earlier than when the predominant direction of growth is vertically downwards. Spread of malignant melanoma is local, lymphatic and haematogenous. Distant metastases commonly occur to the lungs, liver and brain.

The lesion should be completely excised with a wide margin of normal skin. The degree of spread of the tumour should be staged by computed tomography (CT) or MRI scanning. She should be referred to a specialist unit for consideration of radical lymph-node dissection and chemotherapy.

> **🔑 KEY POINTS**
>
> - Melanoma should be suspected if a lesion appears which is black, irregular and bleeding.
> - Fifty per cent of melanomas develop from a pre-existing melanocytic naevus.
> - It should be removed promptly with adequate margins of excision because of the risk of distant metastases.

CASE 31

A 32-year-old woman is admitted as an emergency under the surgical team with acute colicky abdominal pain associated with vomiting and constipation. The pain has developed rapidly over the past 48 hours. She also complains of the development of weakness affecting her arms and legs. She has become extremely agitated and claims to be hearing voices talking about her. She has no significant past medical history. Her father died aged 38 in a psychiatric hospital. She works as a librarian. She is a non-smoker and drinks 20 units of alcohol per week. Her only medication is the oral contraceptive which she started to take three weeks ago.

On examination, she is agitated. She is febrile, 38.0°C. Her pulse is 140/min regular, blood pressure 180/120, jugular venous pressure not raised, heart sounds normal. Her chest is clear. Her abdomen is generally tender, but with no rigidity and bowel sounds are present. The power in her limbs is globally reduced. Tone is normal. Her reflexes are absent. There is loss of pin prick sensation below the knees. Fundoscopy shows papilloedema. The nursing staff notice the patient's urine is dark, but there is no blood or protein on routine testing. The surgical team order investigations:

INVESTIGATIONS

		Normal
Haemoglobin	13.2 g/dl	(11.7–15.7 g/dl)
White cell count	18.4 × 10⁹/l	(3.5–11.0 × 10⁹/l)
Platelets	321 × 10⁹/l	(150–440 × 10⁹/l)
Sodium	124 mmol/l	(135–145 mmol/l)
Potassium	4.2 mmol/l	(3.5–5.0 mmol/l)
Urea	6.2 mmol/l	(2.5–6.7 mmol/l)
Creatinine	112 μmol/l	(70–120 μmol/l)
Glucose	4.6 mmol/l	(4.0–6.0 mmol/l)
Albumin	38 g/l	(35–50 g/l)
Bilirubin	15 μmol/l	(3–17 μmol/l)
Alanine transaminase (ALT)	185 IU/l	(5–35 IU/l)
Alkaline phosphatase	90 IU/l	(30–300 IU/l)

Chest X-ray clear; abdominal X-ray no dilated bowel loops
ECG, sinus tachycardia

QUESTIONS

- What is the diagnosis in this patient?
- How would you investigate and manage this patient?

ANSWER 31

The combination of neuropsychiatric symptoms with acute abdominal pain suggest the unusual condition of **acute intermittent porphyria** in this woman. The positive family history and urine which turns dark on standing are also features of this condition. This most severe type of porphyria is due to an abnormality of porphobilinogen deaminase in the haem biosynthetic pathway. It is an autosomal dominant condition which occurs mainly in young adults and is commoner in women. Peripheral neuropathy complicates about two-thirds of acute porphyria attacks. Weakness of trunk muscles can cause respiratory failure. Grand mal seizures can occur in acute attacks. Sinus tachycardia and systemic hypertension are due to damage to the autonomic nervous system. Attacks may be triggered by drugs (barbiturates, sulphonamides, anticonvulsants, oral contraceptives) as in this case, alcohol, starvation, infection, and pregnancy. A neutrophil leukocytosis and elevated alanine transaminase (ALT) are common as in this woman. Hyponatraemia is due to the associated syndrome of inappropriate antidiuretic hormone (SIADH) secretion.

Unusual non-surgical causes of acute abdominal pain include hypercalcaemia, familial Mediterranean fever, systemic lupus erythematosus, lead poisoning, an abdominal crisis of tabes dorsalis, distended liver (for example due to tricuspid regurgitation), diabetic ketoacidosis and herpes zoster before development of the tell-tale vesicular rash. Myocardial and pleural pathology can also be referred to the abdomen.

An acute attack can be diagnosed by detecting excess urinary porphobilinogen (PBG) and 5-aminolaevulinic acid (ALA). Latent cases can be diagnosed by measuring activity in peripheral blood cells of PBG deaminase and ALA synthase. All relatives should be screened.

This attack should be managed by removing any precipitating factor (stopping the oral contraceptive), maintaining a high carbohydrate intake, providing analgesia with opiates, treating the hypertension and tachycardia with beta-blockers and psychosis with chlorpromazine. Expert advice should be sought and some centres advocate intravenous haematin to reduce the overproduction of porphyrins.

KEY POINTS

- Not all cases of acute abdominal pain are due to surgical causes.
- Acute porphyria should be suspected if a young person presents with a combined abdominal and neuropsychiatric presentation.

CASE 32

A 72-year-old lady presents to her GP. She has felt non-specifically unwell for about two months. She feels stiff especially in the morning. She is unable to get out of bed by herself and has difficulty lifting her hand to comb her hair. She has also noticed pain in her knees and fingers. She has lost 5 kg in weight, and has developed night sweats. In the last few days she has suffered from a constant severe headache, with pain in her jaw when chewing. She has previously been fit with no significant past medical history. She lives alone. She neither smokes nor drinks alcohol. She is taking no regular medication other than occasional paracetamol which has not helped the headache.

On examination, she has lost weight. She is markedly tender to palpation over parts of her scalp. Examination of her cardiovascular, respiratory and abdominal systems is normal. Power is reduced in the proximal muscles of her arms and legs. Neurological examination is otherwise normal.

INVESTIGATIONS

		Normal
Haemoglobin	10.2 g/dl	(11.7–15.7 g/dl)
Mean cell volume	86 fl	(80–99 fl)
White cell count	13.2 × 10⁹/l	(3.5–11.0 × 10⁹/l)
Platelets	376 × 10⁹/l	(150–440 × 10⁹/l)
Erythrocyte sedimentation rate	90 mm/h	(<10mm/h)
Sodium	140 mmol/l	(135–145 mmol/l)
Potassium	4.7 mmol/l	(3.5–5.0 mmol/l)
Urea	3.8 mmol/l	(2.5–6.7 mmol/l)
Creatinine	108 µmol/l	(70–120 µmol/l)
Glucose	4.8 mmol/l	(4.0–6.0 mmol/l)
Albumin	38 g/l	(35–50 g/l)
Bilirubin	16 µmol/l	(3–17 µmol/l)
Alanine transaminase	85 IU/l	(5–35 IU/l)
Alkaline phosphatase	465 IU/l	(30–300 IU/l)
Creatine kinase	134 IU/l	(25–195 IU/l)

QUESTIONS

- What is the diagnosis?
- How would you investigate and manage this patient?

ANSWER 32

This woman has the typical clinical symptoms of **polymyalgia rheumatica/temporal arteritis**. The onset of symptoms is often dramatic. Patients may present primarily with polymyalgia type symptoms (proximal muscle pain and stiffness) or temporal arteritis symptoms (severe headaches with tenderness over the arteries involved). Patients may have systemic symptoms such as general malaise, weight loss and night sweats. Characteristically, the erythrocyte sedimentation rate (ESR) is very elevated and there is a mild anaemia and leukocytosis. The liver enzymes are often slightly raised. This disease usually occurs in patients over 65 years of age. In polymyalgia, the main symptoms are muscle stiffness and pain which may simulate muscle weakness. The creatine kinase is normal unlike polymyositis.

The diagnosis of polymyalgia rheumatica/temporal arteritis is essentially a clinical diagnosis. A very elevated ESR is useful. A temporal artery biopsy should be performed. However, the histology may be normal because the vessel involvement with inflammation is patchy. Nevertheless, a positive result provides reassurance about the diagnosis and the need for long-term steroids.

This patient has clear evidence of a temporal arteritis and is at risk of irreversible visual loss either due to ischaemic damage to the ciliary arteries causing optic neuritis or central retinal artery occlusion. The patient should immediately be started on high-dose prednisolone (before the biopsy result is available). The steroid dose should be slowly tapered according to clinical features and ESR.

> **!** **ALTERNATIVE DIAGNOSES OF PROXIMAL MUSCLE WEAKNESS AND STIFFNESS**
>
> - Polymyositis
> - Systemic vasculitis
> - Systemic lupus erythematosus
> - Parkinsonism
> - Hypothyroidism/hyperthyroidism
> - Osteomalacia

> **⚷ KEY POINTS**
>
> - Patients with polymyalgia rheumatica have markedly elevated ESR levels.
> - There is a risk of blindness and steroids should be started immediately.

A 34-year-old male accountant comes to the accident & emergency department with acute chest pain. There is a previous history of occasional stabbing chest pain for two years. The current pain had come on 4 hours earlier at 8 pm and has been persistent since then. It is central in position, with some radiation to both sides of the chest. It is not associated with shortness of breath or palpitations. The pain is relieved somewhat by sitting up. Two paracetamol tablets taken earlier at 6 pm did not make any difference to the pain.

The previous chest pain had been occasional, lasting a second or two at a time and with no particular precipitating factors. It has usually been on the left side of the chest although the position had varied.

Two weeks previously he had an upper respiratory-tract infection which lasted 3 – 4 days. This consisted of a sore throat, blocked nose, sneezing and a cough. His wife and two children were ill at the same time with similar symptoms but have been well since then. He has a history of migraine. In the family history his father had a myocardial infarction at the age of 51 years and was found to have a marginally high cholesterol level. His mother and two sisters, aged 36 and 38, are well. After his father's infarct he had his lipids measured; the cholesterol was 5.1 mmol/l (desirable range <5.5 mmol/l). He is a non-smoker who drinks 15 units of alcohol per week.

On examination the pulse rate is 75/min, blood pressure 124/78. His temperature is 37.8°C. There is nothing abnormal to find in the cardiovascular or respiratory systems. A chest X-ray is normal. The haemoglobin and white cell count are normal. The creatine kinase level is slightly raised. Other biochemical tests are normal.

The ECG is shown in Fig 33.1.

QUESTIONS

- What is the diagnosis?
- Should thrombolysis with streptokinase be given?

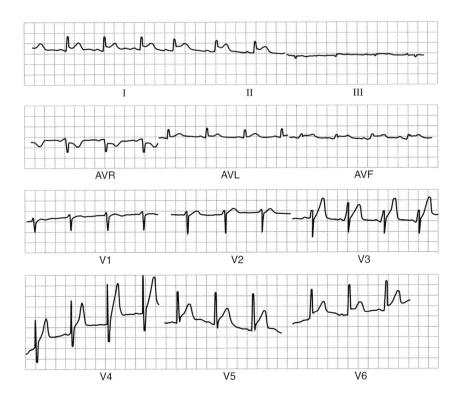

Figure 33.1

ANSWER 33

The previous chest pains lasting a second or two are unlikely to be of any real significance. Cardiac pains, and virtually any other significant pain, lasts longer than this, and stabbing momentary left-sided chest pains are quite common. The positive family history increases the risk of ischaemic heart disease but there are no other risk factors evident from the history and examination. The relief from sitting up leaning forward is typical of pain originating in the pericardium. The ECG shows elevation of the ST segment which is concave upwards, typical of **pericarditis** and unlike the upward convexity found in the ST elevation after myocardial infarction.

The story of an upper respiratory-tract infection shortly before suggests that this may well have a viral aetiology. The viruses commonly involved in pericarditis are Coxsackie B viruses. The absence of a pericardial rub does not rule out pericarditis. Rubs often vary in intensity and may not always be audible. If this diagnosis was suspected, it is often worth listening again on a number of occasions for the rub. Pericarditis often involves some adjacent myocardial inflammation and this could explain the rise in creatine kinase.

Pericarditis may occur as a complication of a myocardial infarction but this tends to occur a day or more later – either inflammation as a direct result of death of the underlying heart muscle or as a later immunological effect (Dressler's syndrome). Pericarditis also occurs as part of various connective-tissue disorders, arteritides, tuberculosis and involvement from other local infections or tumours. Myocardial infarction is not common at the age of 34 years but it certainly occurs. Other causes of chest pain, such as oesophageal pain or musculo-skeletal pain, are not suggested by the history and investigations.

Thrombolysis in the presence of pericarditis carries a slight risk of bleeding into the pericardial space, which could produce tamponade. In this case, the evidence suggests pericarditis and thrombolysis is not indicated. The ECG and enzymes should be followed, the patient re-examined regularly for signs of tamponade (paradoxical pulse with pressure dropping on inspiration, jugular venous pressure rising on inspiration), and analgesics given. In this case, a subsequent rise in antibody titres against Coxsackie virus suggested a viral pericarditis. Symptoms and ECG changes resolved in 4 or 5 days. An echocardiogram did not suggest any pericardial fluid and showed good left ventricular muscle function. The symptoms settled with rest and non-steroidal anti-inflammatory drugs.

KEY POINTS

- ST-segment elevation which is concave upwards is characteristic of pericarditis.
- Viral pericarditis in young people is most often caused by Coxsackie viruses
- Myocarditis may be associated with pericarditis and muscle function should be assessed on echocardiogram and damage from creatine kinase measurements.

CASE 34

A 23-year-old actress presents to her GP complaining that she has not had a menstrual period for five months. She started having periods aged 13 years and previously they have been regular. On direct questioning she states that she has lost 8 kg in weight over the past year although she says her appetite is good. She has had no serious medical illnesses. Although she is an actress, currently she is out of work. She split up from her boyfriend one year ago. She drinks 10 units of alcohol per week and is a non-smoker. She is taking no regular medication.

On examination, she has lost muscle mass especially on her limbs and buttocks. She is 5 ft 9 in tall and weighs only 41 kg. She has excessive hair growth over her cheeks, neck and forearms. Her pulse rate is 52/min regular, blood pressure 96/60. Examination is otherwise normal.

INVESTIGATIONS

		Normal
Haemoglobin	15.2 g/dl	(11.7–15.7 g/dl)
Mean cell volume	84 fl	(80–99 fl)
White cell count	4.1 × 10⁹/l	(3.5–11.0 × 10⁹/l)
Platelets	365 × 10⁹/l	(150–440 × 10⁹/l)
Sodium	136 mmol/l	(135–145 mmol/l)
Potassium	3.1 mmol/l	(3.5–5.0 mmol/l)
Chloride	90 mmol/l	(95–105 mmol/l)
Bicarbonate	33 mmol/l	(24–30 mmol/l)
Urea	4.2 mmol/l	(2.5–6.7 mmol/l)
Creatinine	62 μmol/l	(70–120 μmol/l)
Glucose	5.6 mmol/l	(4.0–6.0 mmol/l)
Albumin	41 g/l	(35–50 g/l)

QUESTIONS

- What is the clinical diagnosis?
- How should this patient be investigated and managed?

ANSWER 34

This picture of loss of menstruation (secondary amenorrhoea), weight loss and hypokalaemic, hypochloraemic metabolic alkalosis fits well with a diagnosis of **anorexia nervosa**. This is a disorder usually of teenagers or young adults characterized by severe weight loss, a disorder of body image (the patient perceiving themself as being fat despite being objectively thin) and amenorrhoea (or, in men loss of libido or potency). It is commoner in women than men. Often sufferers from this condition work in a profession where personal image is very important (e.g. models, actresses, ballet dancers) and there may be a trigger of an emotional upset such as break-up of a relationship or failure in important examinations. They may abuse purgatives or diuretics or cause self-induced vomiting. Some patients exhibit the bulimic behaviour of recurrent bouts of overeating and self-induced vomiting. Patients often deny that they are ill or that they need medical attention. There is marked wasting with obvious bony prominences. The skin is dry with growth of lanugo hair over the neck, cheeks and limbs as in this woman. There is usually a sinus bradycardia and hypotension. Severe physical complications include proximal myopathy, cardiomyopathy and peripheral neuropathy.

❗ MAJOR CAUSES OF SECONDARY AMENORRHOEA

- Hypothalmic/pituitary pathology, e.g. hypopituitarism, hyperprolactinaemia
- Gonadal failure, e.g. autoimmune ovarian failure, polycystic ovaries
- Adrenal disease, e.g. Cushing's disease
- Thyroid disorders, e.g both hypothyroidism and hyperthyroidism
- Severe chronic illnesses, e.g. cancer, chronic renal failure

A number of interrelated mechanisms cause the metabolic alkalosis in this patient. The vomiting causes a net loss of hydrogen and chloride ions, causing alkalosis and hypochloraemia. The loss of fluid by vomiting leads to a contracted plasma volume with consequent secondary hyperaldosteronism to conserve sodium and water, but with renal loss of potassium, due to its secretion in preference to sodium and the fact that fewer hydrogen ions are available for secretion by the renal tubules. These events combine to give the typical picture of an alkalosis with low chloride and raised bicarbonate in the blood, and urine which contains excess potassium and very little chloride. Measurement of 24 hour urinary chloride excretion is helpful. A low urinary chloride excretion (<10 mmol/day) implies vomiting, whereas higher values suggest diuretic abuse.

This patient should be referred to a unit with a special interest in eating disorders. Other serious physical illnesses should be excluded with the appropriate investigations. Plasma levels of luteinizing hormone (LH), follicle-stimulating hormone (FSH) and oestrogens will be low. Often such patients are admitted for several weeks in an attempt to gain weight. This involves a high calorie diet with support from the medical and nursing team. Supportive psychotherapy tackles the patient's disordered perception of their body image.

A 75-year-old woman presents to the casualty department complaining of an episode of paralysis affecting her right arm and leg. The weakness occurred while she was sitting and resolved completely within 10 min. Her husband has previously noticed that she has had episodes of slurred speech lasting a few minutes. She remembers an episode two months earlier when she sensed darkness coming down over her left eye and lasting for a few minutes. She has had non-insulin dependent diabetes mellitus for six years. She is hypertensive and suffered a myocardial infarction two years previously. She smokes about 20 cigarettes per day and does not drink alcohol. Her medication consists of gliclazide for non-insulin dependent diabetes mellitus and atenolol.

On examination she looks frail. Her nails are tar-stained. A bruit is audible on auscultation over the left carotid artery. Her pulse rate is 88/min irregular and blood pressure 172/94. The apex beat is displaced to the sixth intercostal space, mid-axillary line. Her heart sounds are normal and a grade 3/6 pansystolic murmur is audible. Her dorsalis pedis and posterior tibial pulses are not palpable bilaterally. Examination of her chest and abdomen is normal. Neurological examination demonstrates normal tone, power and reflexes. There is no sensory loss. Fundoscopy is normal.

INVESTIGATIONS

		Normal
Haemoglobin	14.3 g/dl	(11.7–15.7 g/dl)
Mean cell volume	86 fl	(80–99 fl)
White cell count	7.4×10^9/l	($3.5–11.0 \times 10^9$/l)
Platelets	282×10^9/l	($150–440 \times 10^9$/l)
Sodium	136 mmol/l	(135–145 mmol/l)
Potassium	3.9 mmol/l	(3.5–5.0 mmol/l)
Urea	6.4 mmol/l	(2.5–6.7 mmol/l)
Creatinine	76 μmol/l	(70–120 μmol/l)
Glucose	4.8 mmol/l	(4.0–6.0 mmol/l)
Chest X-ray	normal	
ECG	atrial fibrillation	

QUESTIONS

- What is the diagnosis?
- How would you manage this patient?

ANSWER 35

This woman gives a history of transient neurological symptoms with no residual signs. She is having recurrent **transient ischaemic attacks** (TIAs) which by definition resolve completely in less than 24 hours. Two months previous to her admission she had an episode of amaurosis fugax (transient uniocular blindness) which is often described as like a shutter coming down over the visual field of one eye. The TIAs are affecting the left cerebral hemisphere in the area of brain supplied by the left carotid artery causing right-sided weakness and dysarthria. TIAs may be caused by thromboembolism from ulcerated plaques in the carotid arteries or aortic arch, from cardiac sources such as a dilated left atrium and more rarely due to haematological causes such as poly-cythaemia rubra vera, sickle cell disease or hyperviscosity due to myeloma. The ECG shows atrial fibrillation and she has the signs of mitral regurgitation with a pansystolic murmur and displaced apex beat. There are three obvious potential sources for emboli:

- a left carotid artery stenosis (in a correct location to account for the distribution of these TIAs)
- the heart in atrial fibrillation with clinically evident mitral regurgitation
- a previous myocardial infarction with mural thrombosis.

> **!** **MAJOR CAUSES OF TRANSIENT NEUROLOGICAL SYNDROMES**
>
> - Migraine. The aura of migraine is a spreading and slowly intensifying phenom-enon and the symptoms are usually positive (e.g scotomata). The aura is usu-ally followed by a severe headache. However, migraines can be associated with focal neurological deficits, e.g hemiplegia.
> - Focal epilepsy. This also normally causes positive symptoms such as twitching and sensory symptoms which may march up one limb and from one limb to another on the same side.
> - Syncope. Unlike most transient ischaemic attacks there is loss of conscious-ness but there are usually no focal signs. Dizziness often precedes the attack.
> - Space-occupying lesion. A cerebral tumour or abscess can produce fluctuat-ing symptoms and signs. The symptoms are usually more gradual in onset and are often associated with headaches or personality changes.
> - Miscellaneous: hysteria, cervical spondylosis, hypoglycaemia and cataplexy.

This patient should be investigated with a computed tomography (CT) head to exclude a structural space occupying lesion, echocardiography to assess left-atrial size, the mitral valve (to exclude infective valvular vegetations) and to rule out thrombus in the left ventricle related to the previous infarct and a Doppler ultrasound of the carotid arteries. If a critical carotid stenosis (> 70 per cent) is present, carotid endarterectomy should be considered. The patient should be anticoagulated with warfarin because of her atrial fibrillation and carotid stenosis.

CASE 36

A 36-year-old man complained of a sudden onset of right-sided chest pain with shortness of breath. This occurred while sitting at home watching television. The pain was made worse by a deep breath and by coughing. The breathlessness persisted over the 4 hours from its onset to his arrival in the accident & emergency department. He has a slight non-productive cough. There is no relevant previous medical history nor any family history of note. He worked as a cashier in a bank and had returned from a three-week holiday in Australia three weeks previously. He takes paracetamol occasionally for headache.

On examination he has a temperature of 37.4°C, his respiratory rate is 24/min, the jugular venous pressure is raised 3 cm, the blood pressure is 110/64, the pulse rate 128/min. In the respiratory system, expansion is reduced because of pain. Percussion and tactile vocal fremitus are normal and equal. A pleural rub can be heard over the right lower zone posteriorly. There are no other added sounds. Otherwise the examination is normal.

An ECG is shown in Fig. 36.1. Fig 36.2 shows his Chest X-ray.

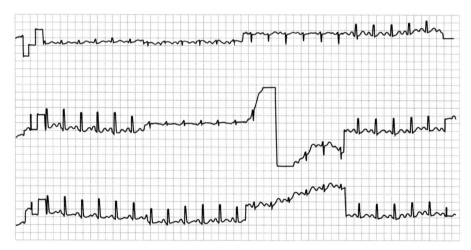

Figure 36.1

QUESTION

- What is the likely diagnosis and how can it be confirmed?

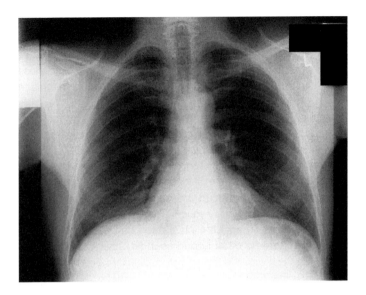

Figure 36.2

ANSWER 36

This man has had a sudden onset of pleuritic pain, breathlessness and cough. The physical signs of tachypnoea, tachycardia, raised jugular venous pressure and pleural rub would fit with a diagnosis of a **pulmonary embolus**.

The differential diagnosis would include pneumonia, pneumothorax and pulmonary embolism. The clinical signs do not suggest pneumothorax or pneumonia. A possible predisposing factor for pulmonary embolism is the history of long aeroplane journeys three weeks earlier. Other predisposing factors such as intravenous drug abuse should be considered. The ECG shows a sinus tachycardia. The often-quoted pattern of S-wave in lead I, Q-wave and T inversion in lead III (S1Q3T3) is not common except with massive pulmonary embolus. Other signs such as transient right ventricular hypertrophy features, P pulmonale and T-wave changes may also occur. The chest X-ray is normal ruling out pneumothorax and lobar pneumonia.

A ventilation–perfusion lung scan was done and showed a typical mismatch with an area at the right base which was ventilated but not perfused. This result had a high probability for a diagnosis of pulmonary embolism. A pulmonary arteriogram is the 'gold standard' for the diagnosis of embolism but is a more invasive test. In cases with a normal chest X-ray and no history of chronic lung disease, equivocal results are less common and it is not usually necessary to go further than the lung scan. In the presence of chronic lung disease such as chronic obstructive pulmonary disease (COPD) or significant asthma, the ventilation–perfusion lung scan is more likely to be equivocal and further tests are more often used. Spiral computed tomography (CT) scan with contrast will show relatively central pulmonary emboli.

A search for a source of emboli with a Doppler of the leg veins may help in some cases and the finding of negative D-dimers in the blood makes intravascular thrombosis and embolism unlikely.

Immediate management should involve heparin as an intravenous infusion or, more simply, as subcutaneous low-molecular-weight heparin. The anticoagulation can then transfer to warfarin, continued in a case like this for six months.

⚲ KEY POINTS

- In the presence of a normal chest X-ray and no chronic lung disease, the ventilation–perfusion lung scan has good sensitivity and specificity.
- The chest X-ray and ECG are often unhelpful in the diagnosis of pulmonary embolism.

A 63-year-old Indian lady is seen by her GP complaining of generalized bony pains and muscle stiffness. Her pains are of a dull ache in quality and worse in her legs. She also complains of difficulty walking, getting up out of chairs and climbing stairs. She is otherwise well. She suffers from long-standing epilepsy for which she takes phenytoin. She is married and lives with her husband and grown-up daughter. She neither smokes nor drinks alcohol.

On examination she looks well. Examination of cardiovascular, respiratory and gastrointestinal systems is normal. Power is reduced symmetrically in her proximal arm and leg muscles. Tone, reflexes, coordination and sensation are normal. She has a waddling gait. The GP organizes blood tests.

INVESTIGATIONS

		Normal
Haemoglobin	12.1 g/dl	(11.7–15.7 g/dl)
Mean cell volume	85 fl	(80–99 fl)
White cell count	8.2×10^9/l	($3.5–11.0 \times 10^9$/l)
Platelets	370×10^9/l	($150–440 \times 10^9$/l)
Erythrocyte sedimentation rate	7 mm/h	(< 10 mm/h)
Sodium	142 mmol/l	(135–145 mmol/l)
Potassium	4.6 mmol/l	(3.5–5.0 mmol/l)
Urea	4.8 mmol/l	(2.5–6.7 mmol/l)
Creatinine	112 μmol/l	(70–120 μmol/l)
Glucose	4.3 mmol/l	(4.0–6.0 mmol/l)
Albumin	38 g/l	(35–50 g/l)
Calcium	1.74 mmol/l	(2.12–2.65 mmol/l)
Phosphate	0.6 mmol/l	(0.8–1.45 mmol/l)
Bilirubin	16 μmol/l	(3–17 μmol/l)
Alanine transaminase	25 IU/l	(5–35 IU/l)
Alkaline phosphatase	480 IU/l	(30–300 IU/l)
Urinalysis	no protein; no blood; no glucose	

QUESTIONS

- What is the diagnosis?
- How would you investigate and manage this patient?

Answer 37

The symptoms and signs are those of a proximal myopathy. In addition, there is bone pain. The investigations show a low calcium and phosphate, and raised alkaline phosphatase. These symptoms and biochemical results suggest **osteomalacia**. This is a condition in which there is inadequate mineralization of bone. There is usually a low serum phosphate and calcium, with a raised alkaline phosphatase. Patients may present with bony pains, particularly in weight-bearing bones. The pain may be severe enough to disturb sleep. There may be difficulty walking or getting out of a chair due to a combination of the pain and associated proximal myopathy. Osteomalacia is due to vitamin D deficiency. Calciferol is absorbed from dietary food and synthesized in the skin. It undergoes 25-hydroxylation in the liver and then 1-hydroxylation in the kidney to 1,25-dihydroxycholecalciferol. This lady has three risk factors for osteomalacia:

- Lack of sun exposure/dark skin.
- Dietary: chapattis reduce absorption of calcium by the gut.
- Phenytoin inhibits 25-hydroxylation of calciferol.

> **!** **DIFFERENTIAL DIAGNOSES OF BONY PAIN AND MUSCLE WEAKNESS**
>
> - Multiple myeloma
> - Bony metastases
> - Paget's disease
> - Chronic renal failure

This patient should have X-rays performed. The radiological hallmark of osteomalacia is the Looser zone. These are translucent ribbon-like bands perpendicular to the surface of the bone, best seen in the long bones, the pubic rami, the ribs and the scapulae. X-ray of the pelvis in this patient shows bilateral Looser's zones in the pubic rami (Fig. 37.1). In another patient, X-ray of the ribs shows multiple Looser's zones, one of which is demonstrated by an arrow (Fig. 37.2). A bone scan may show multiple fractures not seen on the plain films. Bone biopsy is not usually necessary. Her diet should be explored and she should be treated with oral calcium supplements and oral vitamin D.

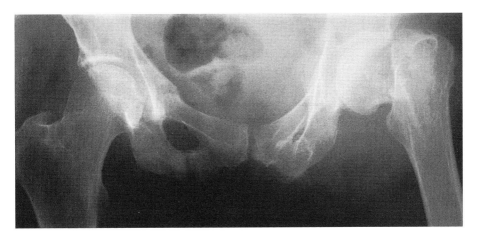

Figure 37.1 X-ray of pelvis. (Reproduced with kind permission of the authors from *Radiology for the MRCP* by Curtis and Whitehouse, published by Arnold in 1998.)

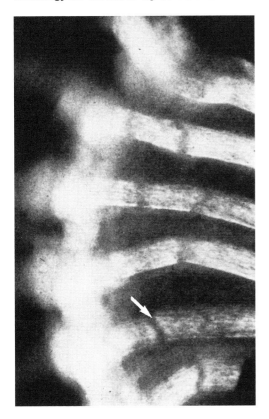

Figure 37.2

105

A 36-year-old man presents to the accident & emergency department at 2 am having vomited blood on two occasions. He had been to an office party the same evening followed by a meal of curry and rice. He began to feel unwell around 11 pm and vomited twice. He vomited up the curry and several pints of lager and initially felt better. However, over the next hour or so he retched violently on several occasions and around 1 am vomited up bright red blood. He says that there was just a small amount of blood on the first occasion but considerably more the second time.

There is no relevant previous medical history or family history. He smokes 10 cigarettes a day, takes occasional marijuana and drinks 2–3 units of alcohol a week.

On examination he seems a little drunk. There is some dried blood around his mouth. The pulse is 98/min and the blood pressure 136/82 lying, with no change on standing. There are no abnormalities on cardiovascular or respiratory examination. In the abdomen there is a little tenderness in the epigastrium.

INVESTIGATIONS

		Normal
Haemoglobin	13.8 g/dl	(13.3–17.7 g/dl)
Mean corpuscular volume (MCV)	87 fl	(80.5–99.7 fl)
White cell count	7.6×10^9/l	($3.9–10.6 \times 10^9$/l)
Platelet count	285×10^9/l	($150–440 \times 10^9$/l)
Sodium	138 mmol/l	(135–145 mmol/l)
Potassium	3.9 mmol/l	(3.5–5.0 mmol/l)
Chloride	99 mmol/l	(95–105 mmol/l)
Urea	5.6 mmol/l	(2.5–6.7 mmol/l)
Creatinine	70 μmol/l	(70–120 μmol/l)
Alkaline phosphatase	184 IU/l	(30–300 IU/l)
Alanine aminotransferase	27 IU/l	(5–35 IU/l)
Gamma-glutamyl transpeptidase	33 IU/l	(11–51 IU/l)

QUESTION

- What is the likely diagnosis?

ANSWER 38

The most likely diagnosis is a tear of the mucosa in the lower oesophagus or upper stomach causing haematemesis (**Mallory–Weiss lesion**). This is produced from the mechanical trauma of violent vomiting or retching. In this case, it is likely to be triggered by an unaccustomed large alcohol intake.

The estimation of blood loss is often difficult from the patient's story. This is a frightening symptom and the amount may be overestimated. The haemoglobin is unlikely to be helpful in an acute bleed. If it were low at this stage it would be more likely to imply chronic blood loss. The first signs of significant blood loss would be likely to be tachycardia and a postural drop in blood pressure. His pulse is fast but this may well be related to anxiety.

Other possible causes of haematemesis are gastritis or peptic ulcer. The story of retching and vomiting of gastric contents with no blood on several occasions before the haematemesis is characteristic of Mallory–Weiss syndrome. This is usually a benign condition which does not need intervention. Definitive diagnosis requires upper gastrointestinal endoscopy but is not always necessary in a typical case. Occasionally the blood loss is more substantial or the split in the wall may be more than just the mucosa leading to perforation.

Management in this case was with intravenous fluid to replace lost volume from vomiting. Blood was taken for blood grouping in case of more substantial haemorrhage but transfusion was not necessary. He was treated with an anti-emetic and an H_2-blocker. The vomiting settled and there was no more bleeding. He decided to indulge less at future Christmas parties.

KEY POINTS

- A history of violent retching or vomiting without blood before haematemesis suggests an upper gastrointestinal mucosal tear.
- It is difficult to be sure of the degree of blood loss in haematemesis because the patient will find it difficult to quantitate the volume of blood and the amount of blood still in the gastrointestinal tract is unknown.

An 81-year-old man is admitted to the casualty department having fallen in his garden and sustained a fractured neck of femur. The orthopaedic surgeons wish to operate on him but they note his abnormal blood results on admission and ask the medical team to review him. His wife explains that he has become increasingly frail over the past six months. He has lost about 8 kg in weight and his appetite is poor. He has complained of worsening pain over his lower back and ribs. He has also told his wife that he feels increasingly lethargic. The patient has had no major previous illnesses. He is a retired solicitor. He is a non-smoker but drinks about 10 units of alcohol per week. He takes only paracetamol for his back pain.

On examination, he looks cachectic. His left leg is shortened and externally rotated. He is also tender to palpation over his T10 vertebra. His conjunctivae are pale. His pulse is 72/min regular, blood pressure 172/88. Physical examination is otherwise normal.

◥ BLOOD TESTS

		Normal
Haemoglobin	6.6 g/dl	(13.3–17.7g/dl)
Mean cell volume	87 fl	(80–99 fl)
White cell count	6.6 × 10⁹/l	(3.9–10.6 × 10⁹/l)
Platelets	112 × 10⁹/l	(150–440 × 10⁹/l)
Erythrocyte sedimentation rate	94mm/h	(< 10 mm/h)
Sodium	135 mmol/l	(135–145 mmol/l)
Potassium	4.7 mmol/l	(3.5–5.0 mmol/l)
Urea	18.2 mmol/l	(2.5–6.7 mmol/l)
Creatinine	294 µmol/l	(70–120 µmol/l)
Calcium	3.14 mmol/l	(2.12–2.65 mmol/l)
Phosphate	1.3 mmol/l	(0.8–1.45 mmol/l)
Total protein	85 g/l	(60–80 g/l)
Albumin	38 g/l	(35–50 g/l)
Bilirubin	12 µmol/l	(3–17 µmol/l)
Alanine transaminase	18 IU/l	(5–35 IU/l)
Alkaline phosphatase	253 IU/l	(30–300 IU/l)
Urinalysis	no protein; no blood	

QUESTIONS

- What is the likely diagnosis?
- What are the major differential diagnoses of causes of fractures?
- How would you investigate and manage this patient?

ANSWER 39

This man has presented with a fracture but his elevated erythrocyte sedimentation rate (ESR), hypercalcaemia and renal impairment are suggestive of **multiple myeloma**. Myeloma is a plasma cell neoplasm occurring mainly in later life producing increased quantities of a gamma globulin from the abnormal clone of plasma cells. It can present with vague symptoms of ill-health, bony pains, increased susceptibility to infections, bleeding complications or renal failure. His raised total protein level with normal albumin implies the presence of a paraprotein. As there is little osteoblastic activity the alkaline phosphatase is normal. This patient's anaemia is due to internal blood loss from his hip fracture, marrow infiltration and renal failure. His thrombocytopenia is due to marrow infiltration.

❗ CAUSES OF SUSCEPTIBILITY TO FRACTURES

- Osteoporosis
- Hyperparathyroidism
- Metastatic carcinoma (especially breast, bronchus, prostate, kidney and thyroid)
- Leukaemia

To confirm the diagnosis, three investigations should be ordered:

1. Serum protein electrophoresis will demonstrate a paraprotein and reduced levels of all immunoglobulin classes (immune paresis). Urinary electrophoresis will detect light chains. These may not be detected by urine dipsticks but will give a positive reaction with sulphasalicylic acid.
2. Bone marrow. The presence of > 10–15 per cent plasma cells indicates myeloma.
3. Radiological skeletal survey. In patients with myeloma there may be numerous punched out lesions in the skull (see Fig. 39.1), vertebral column, ribs, pelvis and long bones. Bone scan is less helpful in detecting myeloma lesions than secondary deposits from carcinoma because of the lack of osteoblastic activity.

This man's hypercalcaemia should be treated with a forced saline diuresis and bisphosphonates. He should be transfused, taking care not to precipitate pulmonary oedema. The haematologists should decide whether chemotherapy is appropriate. The surgeons should operate on his fracture and his healing might benefit from local radiotherapy.

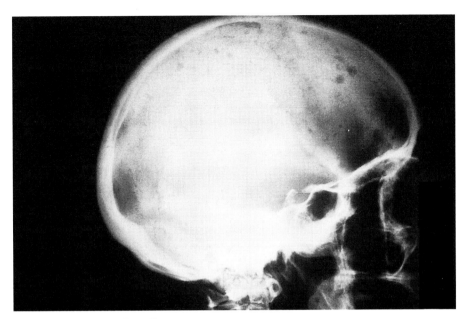

Figure 39.1 X-ray of skull

- Myeloma is a common cause of pathological fractures in the elderly.
- Myeloma deposits produce little osteoblastic reaction so the alkaline phosphatase is often normal and a bone scan does not show hot spots of increased uptake.

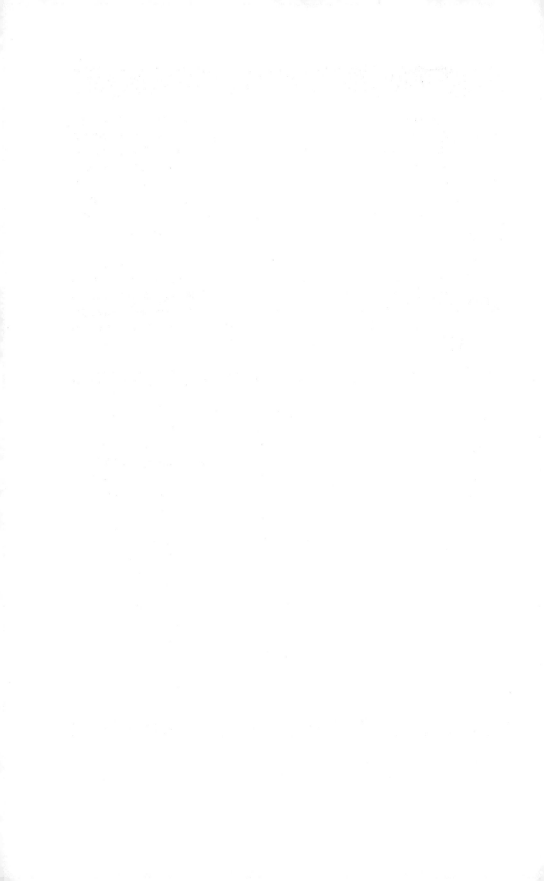

CASE 40

A 78-year-old woman is investigated by her GP for increasing tiredness which has developed over the past six months. She has lost her appetite and feels constantly nauseated. She has lost about 8 kg in weight over the past six months. For the last four weeks she has also complained of generalized itching and cramps. She has been hypertensive for 20 years and has been on antihypertensive medication for that time. She has had two cerebrovascular accidents which have limited her mobility. She is Afro-caribbean having emigrated to the UK in the 1960s. She lives alone but uses a Meals on Wheels service and goes to a day hospital twice a week. She has no family members in the UK.

On examination, her conjunctivae are pale. Her pulse is 88/min regular, blood pressure 190/110; mild pitting oedema of her ankles is present. Otherwise, examination of her cardiovascular and respiratory systems is normal. Neurological examination shows a left upper motor neurone facial palsy with mild weakness and increased reflexes in the left arm and leg. She is able to walk with a stick. Fundoscopy shows arteriovenous nipping and increased tortuosity of the arteries.

INVESTIGATIONS

		Normal
Haemoglobin	7.2 g/dl	(11.7–15.7 g/dl)
Mean cell volume	84 fl	(80–99fl)
White cell count	6.3×10^9/l	($3.5–11.0 \times 10^9$/l)
Platelets	294×10^9/l	($150–440 \times 10^9$/l)
Sodium	136 mmol/l	(135–145 mmol/l)
Potassium	4.8 mmol/l	(3.5–5.0 mmol/l)
Urea	46.2 mmol/l	(2.5–6.7 mmol/l)
Creatinine	769 μmol/l	(70–120 μmol/l)
Glucose	4.1 mmol/l	(4.0–6.0 mmol/l)
Albumin	37 g/l	(35–50 g/l)
Calcium	1.94 mmol/l	(2.12–2.65 mmol/l)
Phosphate	3.4 mmol/l	(0.8–1.45 mmol/l)
Bilirubin	15 μmol/l	(3–17 μmol/l)
Alanine transaminase	23 IU/l	(5–35 IU/l)
Alkaline phosphatase	423 IU/l	(30–300 IU/l)
Urinalysis	+ protein; + blood	
Blood film	normochromic, normocytic anaemia	

QUESTIONS

- What is the diagnosis?
- How would you investigate and manage this patient?

ANSWER 40

This patient presents with the typical symptoms of **end-stage renal failure**, namely anorexia, nausea, weight loss, fatigue, pruritus and cramps.

The elevated urea and creatinine levels confirm renal failure but do not distinguish between acute and chronic renal failure. Usually, in the former, there is either evidence of a systemic illness or some other obvious precipitating cause (e.g. nephrotoxic drugs/hypotension), whereas in the latter there is a prolonged history of general malaise. In this patient, anaemia and hyperparathyroidism (raised alkaline phosphatase) are features indicating chronicity of the renal failure. The normochromic, normocytic anaemia is predominantly due to erythropoietin deficiency (the kidney is the major source of erythropoietin production). Hyperparathyroidism is a result of elevated serum phosphate levels due to decreased renal clearance of phosphate and reduced vitamin D levels (the kidney is the site of hydroxylation of 25-hydroxycholecalciferol to the active form 1,25-dihydroxycholecalciferol). A hand X-ray showing the typical appearances of hyperparathyroidism (erosion of the terminal phalanges and subperiosteal erosions of the radial aspects of the middle phalanges), implying long-standing renal failure can be helpful in distinguishing chronic and acute renal failure.

Renal ultrasound is the essential investigation. Ultrasound will accurately size the kidneys, and identify obvious causes for renal failure such as polycystic kidney disease or obstruction causing bilateral hydronephrosis. Asymmetrically sized kidneys suggest reflux nephropathy or renovascular disease. In this case, ultrasound showed two small (8 cm) echogenic kidneys consistent with long-standing renal failure. A renal biopsy in this case is not appropriate as biopsies of small kidneys have a high incidence of bleeding complications and the sample obtained would show extensive glomerular and tubulo-interstitial fibrosis with no clue as to the original disease. The original disease may have been some form of chronic glomerulonephritis such as IgA nephropathy, or a result of her essential hypertension. Afro-caribbeans are more prone to develop hypertensive renal failure than other racial groups.

Antihypertensive medication is needed to treat her blood pressure adequately, oral phosphate binders and vitamin D preparations to control her secondary hyperparathyroidism, and erythropoietin injections to treat her anaemia. The case raises the dilemma of whether dialysis is appropriate in this patient. Hospital-based haemodialysis or home based peritoneal dialysis are the options available. Her age precludes renal transplantation. The pros and cons of dialysis need to be discussed with the patient, and a multidisciplinary meeting of all her carers (GP, nurses, social workers) should be held.

KEY POINTS

- Patients are often symptomatic with renal failure only when their glomerular filtration rate (GFR) is < 15 ml/min, and thus may present with end-stage renal failure.
- Renal ultrasound visualizing small kidneys is the most useful investigation in helping to confirm that the renal failure is chronic.

A 56-year-old office manager presents to her GP complaining of increasing tiredness over the past few months. She feels depressed, and her husband has noticed her altered mood. She is sleeping poorly and tends to wake up early but denies any suicidal ideas. She also complains of mild nausea and constipation, and notices that she has been more thirsty and passing urine more often. Her legs also ache. She has had two episodes of renal colic in the past three years. She has no significant past medical history. She is married and has three grown up children. She is a non-smoker and drinks 15 units of alcohol per week. She is on no medication.

On examination, the patient appears to have a rather flat emotional appearance with a poverty of facial expression. Her pulse is 76/min, blood pressure 168/94, jugular venous pressure not raised, heart sounds normal with no peripheral oedema. Examination of her respiratory, abdominal and neurological systems is normal. The GP ordered blood tests.

INVESTIGATIONS

		Normal
Haemoglobin	14.2 g/dl	(11.7–15.7 g/dl)
White cell count	7.1×10^9/l	($3.5–11.0 \times 10^9$/l)
Platelets	332×10^9/l	($150–440 \times 10^9$/l)
Sodium	137 mmol/l	(135–145 mmol/l)
Potassium	4.2 mmol/l	(3.5–5.0 mmol/l)
Urea	6.2 mmol/l	(2.5–6.7 mmol/l)
Creatinine	112 μmol/l	(70–120 μmol/l)
Glucose	4.6 mmol/l	(4.0–6.0 mmol/l)
Albumin	38 g/l	(35–50 g/l)
Calcium	3.25 mmol/l	(2.12–2.65 mmol/l)
Phosphate	0.8 mmol/l	(0.8–1.45 mmol/l)
Bilirubin	15 μmol/l	(3–17 μmol/l)
Alanine transaminase	23 IU/l	(5–35 IU/l)
Alkaline phosphatase	323 IU/l	(30–300 IU/l)
Urinalysis	no protein; no blood	

QUESTIONS

- What is the likely explanation for this presentation?
- How would you investigate and manage this patient?

ANSWER 41

This patient has typical symptoms of hypercalcaemia, namely nausea, vomiting, fatigue, constipation, renal colic, bony pain and mood disturbance (most easily remembered as 'moans, stones, bones and groans'!). Other features sometimes seen are proximal myopathy, dyspepsia due to peptic ulceration and back pain due to chronic pancreatitis.

! MAJOR CAUSES OF HYPERCALCAEMIA

- Primary hyperparathyroidism (usually a single benign adenoma)
- Carcinoma with skeletal metastases
- Carcinoma without skeletal metastases (ectopic PTH secretion)
- Myeloma
- Vitamin D intoxication
- Sarcoidosis
- Milk-alkali syndrome
- Thyrotoxicosis
- Prolonged immobility

In this case, the low plasma phosphate level suggests that the cause is excessive parathyroid hormone (PTH) secretion leading to reduced phosphate reabsorption by the renal tubules. In patients with bony metastases, both calcium and phosphate are elevated. In primary hyperparathyroidism the alkaline phosphatase is normal or only slightly raised, whereas in malignancy it is often very high. A further clue that primary hyperparathyroidism rather than malignancy is the cause in this patient is the history of renal calculi suggesting that the hypercalcaemia is chronic. The PTH level was raised in this patient confirming the diagnosis of **primary hyperparathyroidism**. In primary hyperparathyroidism, the PTH levels are inappropriately high for the prevailing calcium level (which may mean a high calcium and normal PTH). In all other cases of hypercalcaemia, the PTH level is suppressed.

Bone X-rays should be performed to exclude metastases and provide evidence of parathyroid bone disease (radiographic evidence is unusual in primary but common in the secondary hyperparathyroidism of chronic renal failure). A chest X-ray helps to exclude bronchial malignancy and sarcoidosis. An electrophoretic strip should be ordered to exclude myeloma. The parathyroid glands may be imaged either by ultrasound or by nuclear medicine scanning. In this patient, a parathyroid scan (using MIBI) was performed, (Fig. 41.1) MIBI is taken up by normal thyroid and parathyroid adenoma tissue at 15 min. At 4 hours, only the parathyroid adenoma is visible (arrow).

The definitive treatment for this patient is surgical removal of the parathyroid adenoma. Her hypercalcaemia has not caused volume depletion or renal failure and therefore treatment is not an emergency. However in the presence of hypovolaemia, the patient should be aggressively hydrated with normal saline and a diuresis maintained with frusemide. Bisphophonates and calcitonin can be used to lower the plasma calcium temporarily.

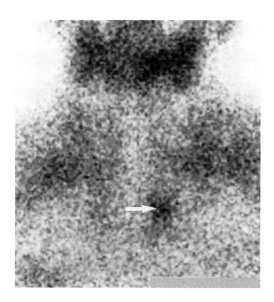

Figure 41.1 Parathyroid scan

A 62-year-old man is admitted to hospital with chest pain. The pain is in the centre of the chest and has lasted for 3 hours by the time of his arrival in the accident & emergency department. The chest pain is central and radiated to the jaw and left shoulder. He felt sick at the same time. He has a history of chest pain on exercise which has been present for six months. He smokes 10 cigarettes each day and does not drink alcohol. He has been treated with aspirin and with β-blockers regularly for the last two years and has been given a glyceryl trinitrate spray to use as needed. This turns out to be two or three times a week. His father died of a myocardial infarction aged 66 years and his 65-year-old brother had a coronary artery bypass graft four years ago.

He has no other previous medical history. He works as a security guard.

On examination he was sweaty and in pain but had no abnormalities to find in the cardiovascular or respiratory systems. His blood pressure was 138/82 and his pulse rate was 110/min and regular. His ECG is shown in Fig. 42.1.

He was given analgesia and streptokinase intravenously and his aspirin and β-blocker were continued. His pain settled and after 2 days he began to mobilize. On the fourth day after admission, he became more unwell.

On examination, now his jugular venous pressure is raised to 6 cm above the manubriosternal angle. His blood pressure is 102/64, pulse rate is 106/min and regular. His temperature is 37.8°C. On auscultation of the heart, there is a loud systolic murmur heard all over the praecordium. In the respiratory system, there are late inspiratory crackles at the lung bases and heard up to the mid-zones. There are no new abnormalities to find elsewhere on examination. His chest X-ray is shown in Fig 42.2.

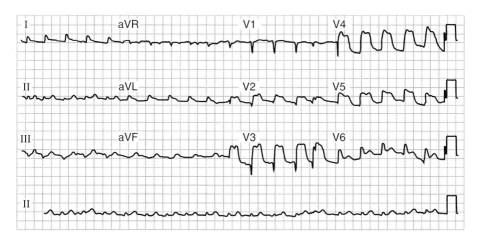

Figure 42.1

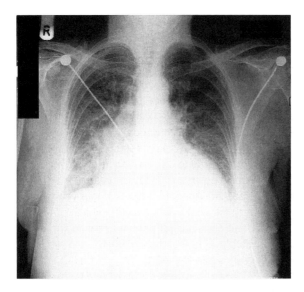

Figure 42.2

- What is the likely diagnosis?
- How might this be confirmed?

Answer 42

This 62-year-old man had an **anteroseptal myocardial infarction** indicated by Q-waves in V2 and V3 and raised ST segments in V2, V3, V4 and V5. He became unwell suddenly 4 days later having had no initial problems. The late inspiratory crackles are typical of pulmonary oedema and the chest X-ray confirms this showing upper-lobe blood diversion and an alveolar filling pattern of shadowing in the lung fields.

The problems likely to occur at this time and produce shortness of breath are a further myocardial infarction, arrhythmias, rupture of the chordae tendinae of the mitral valve, perforation of the intraventricular septum or even the free wall of the ventricle and pulmonary emboli. The first four of these could produce pulmonary oedema and a raised jugular venous pressure as in this man. Pulmonary embolism would be compatible with a raised jugular venous pressure but not the findings of pulmonary oedema on examination and X-ray.

Acute mitral regurgitation from chordal rupture and ischaemic perforation of the interventricular septum both produce a loud pansystolic murmur. The site of maximum intensity of the murmur may differ being apical with chordal rupture and at the lower left sternal edge with ventricular septal defect but this differentiation may not be possible with a loud murmur. The differentiation can be made by echocardiography.

The management of acute ventricular septal defect or chordal rupture would be similar and should involve consultation with the cardiac surgeons. When these lesions produce haemodynamic problems, as in this case, surgical repair is needed either acutely if the problem is very severe or after stabilization with antifailure treatment or even counterpulsation with an aortic balloon pump. Milder degrees of failure with a pansystolic murmur may occur when there is ischaemia of the papillary muscles of the mitral valve. This is managed with antifailure treatment, not surgical intervention, and can be differentiated by echocardiography.

KEY POINTS

- The cause of breathlessness after myocardial infarction needs careful evaluation to determine the cause.
- The signs of ischaemic ventricular septal defect and mitral regurgitation due to chordal rupture after myocardial infarction may be very difficult to differentiate.

An 82-year-old man is sent up to the accident & emergency department by his GP. He is complaining of weakness and general malaise. He has complained of general pains in the muscles and he also has some pains in the joints, particularly the elbows, wrists and knees. Three weeks earlier, he fell and hit his leg and has some local pain related to this.

He is a non-smoker who does not drink any alcohol and has not been on any medication. Twelve years ago he had a myocardial infarction and was put on a beta blocker but he has not had a prescription for this in the last six years. Twenty years ago he had a cholecystectomy. He used to work as a labourer until his retirement at the age of 63 years.

He lives alone in a second-floor flat. His wife died five years ago. He has one son who lives in Ireland and whom he has not seen for three years.

On examination, he is tender over the muscles around his limb girdles and there is a little tenderness over the elbows, wrists and knees. The mouth looks normal except that his tongue appears rather smooth. He has no teeth and has lost his dentures. There are no other abnormalities to find in the cardiovascular, respiratory or alimentary systems. In the legs, he has a superficial laceration on the front of the right shin. This is oozing blood and has not healed. There is a petechial rash on some areas of the legs. There are some larger areas of bruising on the arms and the legs which he says have not been associated with any trauma.

BLOOD TESTS

		Normal
Haemoglobin	10.1 g/dl	13.7–17.7 g/dl
Mean corpuscular volume (MCV)	74 fl	80.5–99.7 fl
White cell count	7.9×10^9/l	$3.9–10.6 \times 10^9$/l
Neutrophils	6.3×10^9/l	$1.8–7.7 \times 10^9$/l
Lymphocytes	1.2×10^9/l	$1.0–4.8 \times 10^9$/l
Platelet count	334×10^9/l	$150–440 \times 10^9$/l

QUESTIONS

- What essential area of the history is not covered above?
- What is the likely diagnosis?

ANSWER 43

A dietary history is an essential part of any history and is particularly important here where a number of features point towards a possible nutritional problem. He has been a widower for five years with no family support. He lives alone on a second-floor flat which may make it difficult for him to get out. He has lost his dentures which is likely to make it difficult for him to eat.

He has a petechial rash which could be related to coagulation problems but the platelet count is normal. It would be important to examine the rash carefully to see if it is distributed around the hair follicles. A number of the features suggest a possible diagnosis of **scurvy** from vitamin C deficiency. Body stores of vitamin C are sufficient to last two to three months. The rash, muscle and joint pains and tenderness, poor wound healing and microcytic anaemia are all features of scurvy. The classic feature of bleeding from the gums would not be present in an edentulous patient.

Plasma measurements of vitamin C are difficult because of the wide range in normal subjects. In this patient, replacement with ascorbic acid orally cleared up the symptoms within two weeks. It would be important to look for other nutritional deficiencies in this situation and to make arrangements to ensure that the situation did not recur after his discharge from hospital.

✎ KEY POINTS

- A nutritional history should be part of any clinical assessment, particularly in the elderly.
- Vitamin deficiencies can occur in patients on a poor diet in the absence of any problem with malabsorption.

CASE 44

A 28-year-old teacher goes to her GP complaining of increased irritability and anxiety. Her change in personality has been noticed by her husband and colleagues at work. She feels constantly restless and has difficulty concentrating on a subject for more than a few moments. Her increased anxiety has developed over the past three months. She has lost 6 kg in weight despite a healthy appetite. She has also noticed an increased frequency of bowel movements. Her periods have become lighter and shorter. She feels extremely tired, sweats profusely and cannot tolerate hot weather. She has had no significant illnesses previously. She is married with no children. She is a non-smoker and drinks 10 units of alcohol per week.

On examination she appears agitated and her hands are sweaty and tremulous. Her eyes appear prominent with lid retraction. Her pulse is 104, regular and blood pressure 130/70. Examination is otherwise normal. Investigations are organized by her GP.

INVESTIGATIONS

		Normal
Haemoglobin	13.2 g/dl	(11.7–15.7 g/dl)
White cell count	4.7 × 10⁹/l	(3.5–11.0 × 10⁹/l)
Platelets	262 × 10⁹/l	(150–440 × 10⁹/l)
Sodium	144 mmol/l	(135–145 mmol/l)
Potassium	4.8 mmol/l	(3.5–5.0 mmol/l)
Bicarbonate	22 mmol/l	(24–30 mmol/l)
Urea	6.2 mmol/l	(2.5–6.7 mmol/l)
Creatinine	88 μmol/l	(70–120 μmol/l)
Glucose	4.2 mmol/l	(4.0–6.0 mmol/l)
Urinalysis	no blood; no protein	

QUESTIONS

- What is the most likely diagnosis?
- How would you manage this patient?

ANSWER 44

Although anxiety might produce some of these symptoms and signs, they fit much better with a diagnosis of **hyperthyroidism**. There was a smooth goitre in the neck and she was found to have a very low thyroxine-stimulating hormone (TSH) level and a high free thyroxine (T4) confirming the diagnosis of hyperthyroidism due to a diffuse toxic goitre (Graves' disease). Hyperthyroidism may mimic an anxiety neurosis with marked restlessness, irritability and distraction. The most helpful discriminatory symptoms are weight loss despite a normal appetite and preference for cold weather. The most helpful signs are goitre, especially with a murmur audible over it, resting sinus tachycardia or atrial fibrillation, tremor and eye signs. Eye signs which may be present include lid retraction (sclera visible below the upper lid), lid lag, proptosis, oedema of the eyelids, congestion of the conjunctiva and ophthalmoplegia. Atypical presentations of thyrotoxicosis include atrial fibrillation in younger patients, unexplained weight loss, proximal myopathy or a toxic confusional state. The very low TSH level suggests a primary thyroid disease rather than overproduction of TSH by the anterior pituitary.

! COMMON CAUSES OF HYPERTHYROIDISM

- Diffuse toxic goitre (Graves' disease)
- Toxic nodular goitre
  - multinodular goitre (Plummer's disease)
  - solitary toxic adenoma
- Overreplacement with thyroxine

Blood should be sent for thyroid-stimulating immunoglobulin which will be detected in patients with Graves' disease. Medical treatment for thyrotoxicosis involves the use of the antithyroid drugs carbimazole or propylthiouracil. These are given for 12–18 months but there is a 50 per cent chance of disease recurrence on stopping the drugs. If this happens radioiodine or surgery is indicated. β-blockers can be used to rapidly improve the symptoms of sympathetic overactivity (tachycardia, tremor) whilst waiting for the antithyroid drugs to act. Radioiodine is effective but there is a high incidence of late hypothyroidism. Surgery is indicated if medical treatment fails, or if the gland is large and compressing surrounding structures. In severe exophthalmos there is a risk of corneal damage and ophthalmological advice should be sought. High-dose steroids, lateral tarsorrhaphy or orbital decompression may be needed.

✎ KEY POINTS

- Thyrotoxicosis may be difficult to differentiate from an anxiety state.
- The commonest causes of hyperthyroidism are Graves' disease or a toxic nodular goitre.

CASE 45

A 24-year-old man presents to his GP with a fever. This has been present on and off for 3 days. On the first day he felt a little shaky but by the third day he felt very unwell with the fever and had a feeling of intense cold with generalized shaking at the same time. He felt very sweaty. The whole episode lasted for 2½ hours and he felt drained and unwell afterwards. He felt off his food.

There was a previous history of hepatitis four years earlier and he had glandular fever at the age of 18 years. He smokes 15–20 cigarettes each day and occasionally smokes marijhuana. He denies any intravenous drug abuse. He drinks around 14 units of alcohol each week. He has taken no other medication except for malaria prophylaxis. He denies any homosexual contacts. He has had a number of heterosexual contacts each year but says that all had been protected intercourse. He had returned from Nigeria three weeks earlier and was finishing off his prophylactic malaria regime. He had been in Nigeria for six weeks as part of his job working for an oil company and had no illnesses while he was there.

On examination he looks unwell. His pulse is 94/min, blood pressure 118/72. There are no heart murmurs. There are no abnormalities to find in the respiratory system. In the abdomen there is some tenderness in the left upper quadrant of the abdomen. There are no enlarged lymph nodes.

INVESTIGATIONS

		Normal
Haemoglobin	11.1 g/dl	13.7–17.7 g/dl
Mean corpuscular volume (MCV)	97 fl	80.5–99.7 fl
White cell count	9.4×10^9/l	$3.9–10.6 \times 10^9$/l
Neutrophils	6.3×10^9/l	$1.8–7.7 \times 10^9$/l
Lymphocytes	2.9×10^9/l	$1.0–4.8 \times 10^9$/l
Platelet count	112×10^9/l	$150–440 \times 10^9$/l
Sodium	134 mmol/l	135–145 mmol/l
Potassium	4.8 mmol/l	3.5–5.0 mmol/l
Urea	4.2 mmol/l	2.5–6.7 mmol/l
Creatinine	74 μmol/l	70–120 μmol/l
Alkaline phosphatase	76 IU/l	30–300 IU/l
Alanine aminotransferase	33 IU/l	5–35 IU/l
Gamma-glutamyl transpeptidase	42 IU/l	11–51 IU/l
Bilirubin	28 μmol/l	3–17 μmol/l
Glucose	4.5 mmol/l	4.0–6.0 mmol/l
Urine	no protein, blood, sugar	

QUESTIONS

- What abnormalities are present in the blood film?
- What is the most likely diagnosis?
- What would be the appropriate management?

ANSWER 45

There is a raised bilirubin with normal liver enzymes, a mild anaemia with a high normal mean corpuscular volume and a low platelet count. This makes a haemolytic anaemia likely. The recent travel to Nigeria raises the possibility of an illness acquired there. The commonest such illness causing a fever in the weeks after return is **malaria**. The incubation period is usually 10–14 days. The mild haemolytic anaemia with a low platelet count would be typical findings. Enlargement of liver and spleen may occur in malaria.

The diagnosis should be confirmed by appropriate expert examination of a blood film.

The most important feature in this 24-year-old man is the fever with what sound like rigors. He has no other specific symptoms. He looks unwell with a tachycardia and some tenderness in the left upper quadrant which could be related to splenic enlargement.

Malaria prophylaxis is often not taken regularly. Even when it is, it does not provide complete protection against malaria which should always be suspected in circumstances such as those described here. The risk might be assessed further by finding which parts of Nigeria he spent his time in and whether he remembered mosquito bites. Measures to avoid mosquito bites such as nets, insect repellants and suitable clothing are an important part of prevention.

He has no history of intravenous drug abuse or recent risky sexual contact to suggest HIV infection although this could not be ruled out. HIV seroconversion can produce a feverish illness but not usually as severe as this. Later in HIV infection an AIDS-related illness would often be associated with a low total lymphocyte count, but this is normal in his case. Other acute viral or bacterial infections are possible but are less likely to explain the abnormal results of some investigations.

The diagnostic test for malaria is staining of a peripheral blood film with Wright or Giemsa stain. In this case it showed that around 1 per cent of red cells contained parasites. Treatment depends on the likely resistance pattern in the area visited and up-to-date advice can be obtained by telephone from tropical disease hospitals. Falciparum malaria is usually treated with quinine sulphate because of widespread resistance to chloroquine. A single dose of Fansidar (pyrimethamine and sulfadoxine) is given at the end of the quinine course for final eradication of parasites.

In severe cases hyponatraemia and hypoglycaemia may occur and the sodium here is marginally low. Most of the severe complications are associated with *Plasmodium falciparum* malaria. They include cerebral malaria, lung involvement, severe haemolysis and acute renal failure.

⚓ KEY POINTS

- No prophylactic regime is certain to prevent malaria.
- Treatment should be guided by advice from tropical disease centres (telephone numbers in the *British National Formulary*).
- If the malaria species is unknown or the infection mixed, treat as falciparum malaria

A 27-year-old woman has an eight-year history of abdominal pain and bloating. She has had an irregular bowel habit with periods of increased bowel actions up to four times a day and periods of constipation. Opening her bowels tends to relieve the pain which has been present in both iliac fossae at different times. She had similar problems around the age of 17 years which led to time off school. She thinks that her pains are made worse after eating citrus fruits and after some vegetables and wheat. She has tried to exclude these from her diet with some temporary relief but overall there has been no change in the symptoms over the eight years.

She has a history of occasional episodes of headache which have been diagnosed as migraine and has irregular periods with troublesome period pains but no other relevant medical history. She is a non-smoker who does not drink alcohol. Her paternal grandmother died of carcinoma of the colon aged 64 years. Her parents are alive and well. She works as a secretary.

On examination her heart rate, blood pressure and examination of the cardiovascular and respiratory systems are all normal. She has a palpable, rather tender colon in the left iliac fossa. Her blood count, sedimentation rate, electrolytes and liver function have been done over the last six weeks and are all normal.

One year previously she was seen in a gastroenterology clinic and had a sigmoidoscopy which was normal. She found the procedure very uncomfortable and developed similar symptoms of abdominal pain during the procedure.

She is anxious about the continuing pain but is not keen to have a further endoscopy.

QUESTION

- What is the most likely diagnosis and what investigations should be performed?

ANSWER 46

The pattern of the pain, the absence of physical signs, normal investigations and reproduction of the pain during sigmoidoscopy all make it likely that this is **irritable bowel syndrome** (IBS). In IBS it is common to have a history of other conditions such as migraine and menstrual irregularity. Under the age of 40 years with a history of eight years of similar problems, it would be reasonable to accept the diagnosis and reassure the patient. However, the family history of carcinoma of the colon raises the possibility of a condition such as familial polyposis coli. The family history, the circumstances of the grandmother's death and the patient's feelings about this should be explored further. Anxiety about the family history might contribute to the patient's own symptoms or her presentation at this time. If there are living family members with polyposis coli, DNA probing may be used to identify family members at high risk. If any doubt remains in this woman it would be sensible to proceed to a barium enema or a colonoscopy to rule out any significant problems.

The diagnosis of IBS relies on the exclusion of other significant conditions. In patients under the age of 40 it is usually reasonable to do this on the basis of the history and examination. In older patients, sigmoidoscopy and barium enema or colonoscopy should be performed to rule out colonic malignancy, diverticular disease and inflammatory bowel disease. A plan of investigation and management should be clearly established. The symptoms tend to be persistent and are not helped by repeated normal investigations looking for an underlying cause. Symptoms may be helped by antispasmodic drugs or tricyclic antidepressants.

KEY POINTS

- Irritable bowel syndrome is a common disorder and difficult to treat. Explanation of the condition to the patient is an important part of the management.
- Sigmoidoscopy with air insufflation often reproduces the symptoms of IBS.

A 73-year-old woman presents to the casualty department complaining of increasing breathlessness over the previous 4 days. She has felt unwell for two months and has lost 4 kg in weight. She has had frequent nosebleeds, and over the past few days has coughed up small amounts of fresh blood. She notices that she has been passing less urine in the past few days.

On examination, she is febrile (38.0°C), centrally cyanosed and looks unwell. She has a purpuric rash over her ankles. Her pulse is 104/min regular, blood pressure 120/90. Her jugular venous pressure is not raised. Her heart sounds are normal with no added sounds. Her respiratory rate is 30 breaths/min, expansion is reduced, percussion and tactile vocal fremitus are normal but she has coarse inspiratory crackles throughout both lung fields. Her abdominal and neurological examination is normal.

INVESTIGATIONS

		Normal
Haemoglobin	10.1 g/dl	(11.7–15.7 g/dl)
Mean cell volume	87 fl	(80–99 fl)
White cell count	$17.2 \times 10^9/l$	$(3.5–11.0 \times 10^9/l)$
Platelets	$540 \times 10^9/l$	$(150–440 \times 10^9/l)$
Sodium	137 mmol/l	(135–145 mmol/l)
Potassium	6.6 mmol/l	(3.5–5.0 mmol/l)
Bicarbonate	8 mmol/l	(24–30 mmol/l)
Urea	45.1 mmol/l	(2.5–6.7 mmol/l)
Creatinine	832 μmol/l	(70–120 μmol/l)
Glucose	4.6 mmol/l	(4.0–6.0 mmol/l)
Albumin	32 g/l	(35–50 g/l)
Calcium	2.23 mmol/l	(2.12–2.65 mmol/l)
Phosphate	1.9 mmol/l	(0.8–1.45 mmol/l)
Arterial blood gases (on air)		
pH	7.18	(7.38–7.44)
pCO_2	5.1 kPa	(4.7–6.0 kPa)
pO_2	6.4 kPa	(12.0–14.5 kPa)
Urinalysis	++ protein; +++ blood	
Urine microscopy	>100 red cells; red cell casts; no organisms	
ECG	sinus tachycardia	
Chest X-ray		

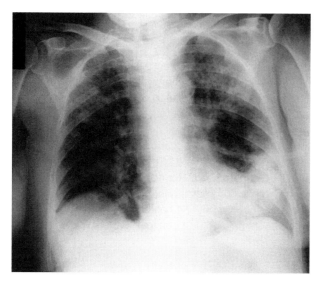

Figure 47.1

- What is the likely diagnosis?
- How would you manage and investigate this patient?

ANSWER 47

This woman has an illness affecting her lungs and kidneys. Her investigations show renal and respiratory failure. Respiratory failure may occur due to fluid overload in renal failure but the findings on examination (normal jugular venous pressure, coarse pan-inspiratory crackles rather than fine, late inspiratory crackles) do not support this. The chest X-ray shows bilateral infiltrates affecting both upper zones and left lower zone (an oxygen mask tubing is visible over the left lung). The purpuric rash and the raised platelet count are typical of an active vasculitis.

> ### ! MAJOR CAUSES OF PULMONARY/RENAL SYNDROME
>
> - Systemic vasculitis e.g. Wegener's granulomatosis, microscopic polyarteritis.
> - Goodpasture's disease (antiglomerular basement-membrane disease and pulmonary haemorrhage)
> - Systemic lupus erythematosus

The history of nosebleeds implying upper respiratory tract involvement suggests that the most likely diagnosis is **Wegener's granulomatosis** rather than microscopic polyarteritis. Both are conditions of small vessel vasculitis and cause a necrotizing glomerulonephritis and pulmonary haemorrhage, and can affect other organs such as the skin, joints, eyes and nervous system. Antiglomerular basement-membrane disease is unlikely in this case as it does not cause a rash. The other principal differential diagnoses of vasculitis include atheroembolic disease, infective endocarditis and meningococcal septicaemia.

This lady needs emergency treatment for her respiratory failure, metabolic acidosis and hyperkalaemia. She requires respiratory support with oxygen treatment. If this does not produce adequate oxygenation mechanical ventilation may need to be considered. Her hyperkalaemia needs emergency treatment with intravenous calcium gluconate and an infusion of dextrose and insulin whilst haemodialysis is being organized.

All patients with acute renal failure should have a renal ultrasound to size the kidneys and rule out obstruction. A renal biopsy in this patient will provide histological confirmation of systemic vasculitis by showing a focal necrotizing glomerulonephritis usually with crescent formation. Biopsy of nasal lesions is often unproductive, showing only necrotic tissue and may delay diagnosis. Blood should be sent for antineutrophil cytoplasmic antibodies which are present in about 90 per cent of untreated cases of small-vessel vasculitis. A gas transfer factor K_{co} will be temporarily increased in this patient because of her acute pulmonary haemorrhage. Red cells in the alveoli take up the carbon monoxide, as well as those in the alveolar capillaries until their haemoglobin is denatured a day or so later. The specific treatment for this lady involves intensive immunosuppression with intravenous methylprednisolone, oral cyclophosphamide and plasma exchange. After the acute-phase, maintenance treatment is oral prednisolone and azathioprine.

An 86-year-old woman is brought in to hospital by ambulance having been found on the floor at home unconscious. Her home help found her when she came in on Monday morning. She was seen last by the home help on the Friday afternoon. She gets out of the house occasionally in the summer but has not left the house over the last two to three months because of arthritis in the hips and the winter weather.

The home help thinks that she has a past history of a hiatus hernia, gallstones, osteoarthritis and non-insulin-dependent diabetes mellitus controlled by diet. She takes some ranitidine for indigestion and co-proxamol (paracetamol and dextro-propoxyphene) for arthritic pains. Her sister says that there is a family history of dia-betes and thyroid trouble. Her GP is contacted by telephone and confirms the med-ication and previous medical history.

On examination she looks pale. She smells of urine. There are no localizing neuro-logical signs. Tendon reflexes are present and equal except the ankle reflexes which are absent. Plantars responses are downgoing. The pupils are equal and reactive and the fundi look normal. The observation chart is completed by the nurse in the accident & emergency department.

INVESTIGATIONS

- Pulse, 82/min
- Blood pressure, 92/56
- Temperature, 35.1°C
- Respiratory rate, 12/min
- Oxygen saturation, 95 per cent breathing air
- Glasgow Coma Scale, 10/15
- Urine on catheterisation; 450 ml volume, sugar +, blood +, no protein

The ECG is shown in Fig. 48.1.

QUESTIONS

- What is the likely cause of the problem?
- What investigations and treatment are indicated?

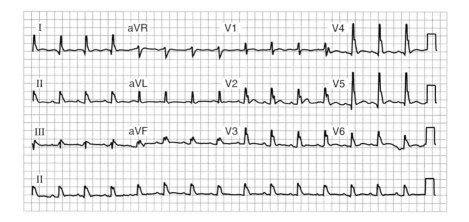

Figure 48.1

ANSWER 48

This woman has been on the floor at home for anything up to 66 hours. There are a number of possible causes for her unconsciousness including a cerebrovascular problem, deliberate or accidental drug overdose (e.g. with the paracetamol/dextropropoxyphene), metabolic or endocrine disturbance or hypothermia.

If this were an overdose of paracetamol/dextropropoxyphene, the pupils might well be small from the synthetic opioid. The slow respiratory rate could be compatible with an opiate excess suppressing ventilation. The oxygen saturation results show that she is oxygenating herself satisfactorily although it would be sensible to perform blood gases to measure the p_aco_2 level. It would be appropriate to measure the paracetamol level in the blood and it would be worth giving the opiate antagonist naloxone if there remained a likelihood of overdose.

Most cerebrovascular problems would be expected to produce some localizing neurological signs on careful examination even in an unconscious patient. There are no such signs here. The absent ankle jerks might be related to her age or diabetes.

She could have hyperosmolar non-ketotic coma detected by a high glucose and evidence of haemoconcentration. The blood glucose should be measured together with electrolytes and haematology but the single + of glucose in the urine makes it unlikely that she has hyperglycaemic coma. Liver function and renal function should be measured.

She has a slow respiratory rate, low blood pressure and an ECG which shows a wide QRS complex. The pulse rate would often be slower than the 82/min in this woman and the ECG may show evidence of a tremor from shivering. The wide complexes on the ECG show an extra deflection at the end of the QRS complex, the J point. This J-wave is characteristic of hypothermia and disappears after rewarming as shown by the subsequent ECG (Fig 48.2). The temperature of 35.1°C does not appear excessively low but this may not be reliable if it has been measured with a normal mercury thermometer. (Mercury thermometers are not reliable at low temperatures.) Indeed, in this case, repeat of the rectal temperature measurement with a low-reading thermometer showed a temperature of 30.6°C.

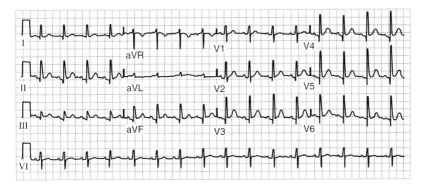

Figure 48.2 ECG of resolved hypothermia

The management of hypothermia in the elderly is gradual rewarming with replacement of fluids by warmed colloids as rewarming takes place. The increase of temperature should be 0.5 to 1°C per hour. If this is not achieved by covering the patient with blankets, then warmed inspired oxygen, warm intravenous fluids, bladder or peritoneal lavage might be considered. Drugs and physical disturbance should be limited since the myocardium is often irritable and susceptible to arrhythmias.

✎ KEY POINTS

- Hypothyroidism should be considered as a possible contributor to hypothermia.
- The diagnosis of hypothermia requires a thermometer capable of reading low temperatures.
- J-waves on the ECG are specific signs of hypothermia.
- Hypothermia in the elderly is treated by gradual rewarming.

CASE 49

A 32-year-old homosexual man had a positive HIV test five years ago. He has been followed up regularly in a genitourinary medicine clinic. For a year or two he took anti-retroviral therapy but has been on no antiretroviral treatment for the last year. His CD4 lymphocyte count has been monitored regularly and fell below 200/mm³ eight months ago. At that time he began regular treatment with co-trimoxazole as prophylaxis against pneumocystis pneumonia. He says that he has taken this regularly. This is his only treatment except for vitamins and homeopathic mixtures.

He began to feel more unwell five weeks ago with increasing lethargy, headaches, sweats and a fever. He began to record his temperature and initially this rose to 38°C on some days. Over the last week it has been up to 38.5 or 39°C most days and he has felt more unwell. He has lost 6 kg in weight over the last month. His bowel motions have been loose and his bowels have been open two or three times a day.

On examination, he looks thin. There are some small lymph nodes palpable in the axillae and supraclavicular areas but the largest is only 1 cm diameter. There is some oral candidiasis.

INVESTIGATIONS

Chest X-ray	normal	
Lumbar puncture and investigation of CSF	normal	
Cryptococcal antigen in the blood	normal	
Toxoplasma antibodies	normal	
Venereal Disease Research Laboratory	normal	

		Normal
Haemoglobin	11.1 g/dl	13.7–17.7 g/dl
Mean corpuscular volume (MCV)	83 fl	80.5–99.7 fl
White cell count	3.8 × 10⁹/l	3.9–10.6 × 10⁹/l
Platelet count	86 × 10⁹/l	150–440 × 10⁹/l
Sodium	137 mmol/l	135–145 mmol/l
Potassium	4.0 mmol/l	3.5–5.0 mmol/l
Urea	4.1 mmol/l	2.3–6.7 mmol/l
Creatinine	72 μmol/l	70–120 μmol/l
Alkaline phosphatase	144 IU/l	30–300 IU/l
Alanine aminotransferase	46 IU/l	5–35 IU/l
Gamma-glutamyl transpeptidase	68 IU/l	11–51 IU/l

QUESTIONS

- What is your interpretation of these findings?
- What are the likely diagnoses?
- What other tests should be performed?

ANSWER 49

The blood results show mild anaemia with a low total white count and low platelets. The liver-function tests are mildly abnormal. In addition, he has a fever and mild bowel upset. He has some general mild lymphadenopathy but this does not appear to be very impressive and might well give no other useful information if biopsied. It should be watched carefully and biopsied if there is further enlargement. The anaemia and low platelets may be part of his HIV disease. The length of the history makes a simple viral or bacterial infection less likely and raises the likelihood of an opportunist pathogen.

With a fever, useful information might be obtained from a bone marrow biopsy and culture including acid-fast bacilli. The stool should be cultured and examined for pathogens. Other possible investigations would be an ultrasound of the liver and a sigmoidoscopy with rectal biopsy for pathogens. The sinuses are another area where infection may be relatively silent in HIV disease. The other important investigations are blood cultures including special cultures for acid-fast bacilli.

In this case the mycobacterial blood cultures were positive and the organism which grew was **Mycobacterium avium complex** (MAC). This can affect any organs and may explain the bone marrow, liver, bowel and lymph-node changes in this man, although other additional pathogens need to be considered.

The differential diagnosis includes bowel pathogens, tuberculosis or more likely with a normal chest X-ray, non-tuberculous mycobacteria such as MAC. Viral infections such as herpes simplex and cytomegalovirus are also likely. Tumours such as lymphoma could also present in this way.

MAC is a difficult organism to treat. Various combinations of antibiotics can be useful in suppressing the manifestations of the disease but they do not usually eradicate the organism permanently. In the USA and some other countries prophylaxis with rifabutin is recommended to prevent MAC disease but this is not widespread practice in the UK and may be no more effective than rifampicin.

KEY POINTS

- Mycobacteria may be cultured from the blood in HIV disease. Special blood culture bottles must be used.
- MAC can be suppressed for a while in AIDS patients but the prognosis at this stage is usually no more than a few months.

CASE 50

A 50-year-old man presents to accident & emergency with acute weakness of both legs. Three weeks prior to his admission he had an upper respiratory-tract infection. Two days before admission he started to develop difficulty walking but he is now completely unable to move his legs below his knees. Both feet are also painful. His bowels and bladder are functioning normally. He has no significant past medical history. He neither smokes nor drinks alcohol and is taking no medication.

On examination, he looks well. His pulse rate is 104/min, and blood pressure 166/102. His jugular venous pressure is not raised and examination of his heart, respiratory and abdominal systems is normal. Neurological examination shows grade 0/5 power below his knees and 1/5 power for hip flexion/extension. His legs are hypotonic. Knee and ankle reflex jerks are absent. There is impaired pin-prick sensation up to the groin and reduced joint position sense and vibration sense in the lower limbs. Examination of his arms is normal.

Initial haematology and biochemistry results are normal. The results of his lumbar puncture are shown.

LUMBAR PUNCTURE

		Normal
CSF	clear	
CSF protein	3.4 g/l	(0.4g/l)
CSF glucose	4 mmol/l	(>70 per cent plasma glucose)
Leukocytes	5/μl	(<5/μl)
Plasma glucose	4.5 mmol/l	
Gram stain	no organisms	

QUESTIONS

- What is the diagnosis?
- What are the major differential diagnoses?
- How would you manage this patient?

ANSWER 50

The most marked features are the loss of power with absent reflexes suggesting a lower motor neurone lesion. The sensory disturbance is less severe and he has a sensory level around L2. This man has **Guillain–Barré syndrome** (acute idiopathic inflammatory polyneuropathy). This disorder is a polyneuropathy which develops usually over two to three weeks, but sometimes more rapidly. It commonly follows a viral infection or *Campylobacter* gastroenteritis and a fever is common. It predominantly causes a motor neuropathy which can either have a proximal, distal or generalized distribution. Distal paraesthesiae and sensory loss are common. Reflexes are lost early. Cranial and bulbar nerve paralysis may occur and can cause respiratory failure. The CSF protein is usually raised, but the cell count is usually normal, although there may be a mild lymphocytosis. The disorder is probably due to a cell-mediated delayed hypersensitivity reaction causing myelin to be stripped off the axons by mononuclear cells.

! DIFFERENTIAL DIAGNOSES OF MOTOR NEUROPATHY

- Guillain–Barré syndrome
- Lead poisoning
- Porphyria
- Diphtheria
- Charcot–Marie–Tooth disease (hereditary motor and sensory neuropathy)
- Poliomyelitis
  An acute-onset neuropathy suggests:
- Guillain–Barre syndrome
- Porphyria
- Malignancy
- Some toxic neuropathies
- Diphtheria
- Botulism

This patient should be referred to a neurologist for further investigation and management. In this patient who presents with weakness and sensory signs, it is important to make sure there is not evidence of spinal cord compression or multiple sclerosis. However, these would tend to cause hypertonia, hyperreflexia and a more distinct sensory level. A MRI of brain and spinal cord should therefore be considered. Nerve-conduction studies will confirm a neuropathy. He should be treated either with plasma exchange or intravenous immunoglobulin. His respiratory function should be monitored with daily spirometry and mechanical ventilation may be necessary. Most patients recover over a period of several weeks.

⚲ KEY POINTS

- Guillain–Barré syndrome presents with predominantly a motor neuropathy although sensory symptoms are usually present.
- There is often a history of an infective illness in the previous three weeks, often *Campylobacter jejuni*.

CASE 51

An 18-year-old girl has a history of repeated chest infections. She had problems with a cough and sputum production in the first two years of life and was labelled as bronchitic. Over the next 14 years she was often 'chesty' and had spent four to five weeks a year away from school. Over the last two years she has developed more problems and was admitted to hospital on three occasions with cough and purulent sputum. On the first two occasions, *Haemophilus influenzae* was grown on culture of the sputum and on the last occasion two months previously *Pseudomonas aeruginosa* was isolated from the sputum at the time of admission to hospital. She is still coughing up sputum. Although she has largely recovered from the infection, her mother is worried and asked for a further sputum to be sent off. The report has come back from the microbiology laboratory showing that there is a scanty growth of *Pseudomonas* on culture of the sputum.

There is no family history of any chest disease. Routine questioning shows that her appetite is reasonable, micturition is normal, bowels tend to be irregular and menstruation started rather late at 15 years.

On examination she is thin, weighing 44 kg and 5 ft 5 in tall. The only finding in the chest is of a few inspiratory crackles over the upper zones of both lungs. Cardiovascular and abdominal examination is normal. The chest X-ray is shown in Fig 51.1.

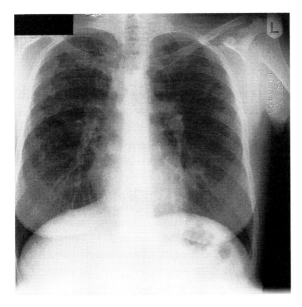

Figure 51.1

QUESTIONS

- What does the X-ray show?
- What is the most likely diagnosis?
- What investigations should be performed?

ANSWER 51

The chest X-ray shows abnormal shadowing in both upper lobes with some ring shadows and tubular shadows representing thickened bronchial walls. These findings would be compatible with a diagnosis of bronchiectasis. The distribution is typical of that found in **cystic fibrosis** where the changes are most evident in the upper lobes. Most other forms of bronchiectasis are more likely to occur in the lower lobes where drainage by gravity is less effective. High-resolution computed tomography (CT) of the lungs is the best way to diagnose bronchiectasis and to define its extent and distribution. In younger and milder cases of cystic fibrosis the predominant organisms in the sputum are *Haemophilus influenzae* and *Staphylococcus aureus*. Later, as more lung damage occurs, *Pseudomonas aeruginosa* is a common pathogen. Once present in the lungs in cystic fibrosis, it is difficult or impossible to remove it completely.

Cystic fibrosis should always be considered when there is a story of repeated chest infections in a young person. Although it presents most often below the age of 20 years, diagnosis may be delayed until the twenties, thirties or even forties in milder cases. Associated problems occur in the pancreas (malabsorption, diabetes), sinuses and liver. It has become evident that some patients are affected more mildly, especially those with the less common genetic variants. These milder cases may only be affected by the chest problems of cystic fibrosis and have little or no malabsorption from the pancreatic insufficiency.

The differential diagnosis in this girl would be other causes of diffuse bronchiectasis such as agammaglobulinaemia or immotile cilia. Respiratory function should be measured to see the degree of functional impairment. Bronchiectasis in the upper lobes may occur in tuberculosis or in allergic bronchopulmonary aspergillosis associated with asthma.

The common diagnostic test for cystic fibrosis is to measure the electrolytes in the sweat where there is an abnormally high concentration of sodium and chloride. At the age of 18, the sweat test may be less reliable. It is more specific if repeated after the administration of fludrocortisone. An alternative would be to have the potential difference across the nasal epithelium measured at a centre with a special interest in cystic fibrosis. Cystic fibrosis has an autosomal recessive inheritance with the commonest genetic abnormality ∆F508 found in 85 per cent of cases. The gene is responsible for the protein controlling chloride transport across the cell membrane. The commoner genetic abnormalities can be identified and the current battery of genetic tests identifies over 95 per cent of cases. However, the absence of ∆F508 and other common abnormalities would not rule out cystic fibrosis related to the less common genetic variants.

In later stages, lung transplantation can be considered. Since the identification of the genetic abnormality, trials of gene-replacement therapy have begun.

✎ KEY POINTS

- Milder forms of cystic fibrosis may present in adolescence and adulthood.
- Milder forms are often related to less common genetic abnormalities.
- A high-resolution CT scan is the best way to detect bronchiectasis and to define its extent.

CASE 52

A 23-year-old Afro-caribbean woman is admitted to the casualty department having had two tonic–clonic generalized seizures. These were witnessed by her mother with whom she lives. Her mother says that her daughter has been behaving increasingly strangely, and has been hearing voices talking about her. She has complained recently of severe headaches. She has recently lost weight and has noticed that her hair has been falling out. She has also complained of night sweats and flitting joint pains affecting mainly the small joints of her hands and feet. She works as a bank clerk. She smokes 5–10 cigarettes per day and consumes about 10 units of alcohol per week. She is taking no regular medication. She has no significant medical or psychiatric history.

On examination, she is drowsy but responsive to pain. There is no neck stiffness. Her scalp hair is thin and patchy. Her temperature is 38.5°C. She has small generalized palpable lymph nodes. Her pulse rate is 104/min regular, blood pressure 164/102. Examination of her cardiovascular, respiratory and abdominal systems is otherwise normal. Neurological examination reveals no focal abnormality and no papilloedema.

INVESTIGATIONS

		Normal
Haemoglobin	7.2 g/dl	(11.7–15.7 g/dl)
Mean cell volume	85 fl	(80–99 fl)
White cell count	2.2 × 10⁹/l	(3.5–11.0 × 10⁹/l)
Platelets	72 × 10⁹/l	(150–440 × 10⁹/l)
Erythrocyte sedimentation rate	90 mm/h	(<10mm/h)
Sodium	136 mmol/l	(135–145 mmol/l)
Potassium	4.2 mmol/l	(3.5–5.0 mmol/l)
Urea	16.4 mmol/l	(2.5–6.7 mmol/l)
Creatinine	176 µmol/l	(70–120 µmol/l)
Glucose	4.8 mmol/l	(4.0–6.0 mmol/l)
Urinalysis	+++ protein; +++ blood	
Urine microscopy	red cells ++; red cell casts present	
Chest X-ray	normal	
ECG	sinus tachycardia	
CT brain	normal	
Lumbar puncture		
Leukocytes	150/µl	(<5/µl)
CSF protein	1.2 g/l	(<0.4g/l)
CSF glucose	4.1 mmol/l	(>70 per cent plasma glucose)
Gram stain	negative	

QUESTIONS

- What is the likely diagnosis?
- How would you investigate and manage this patient?

ANSWER 52

There are a number of important symptoms, particularly the generalized seizures, auditory hallucinations, fever, arthralgia and alopecia. The investigations show low haemoglobin, white cells and platelets with impaired renal function and blood, protein and cells in the urine. The CSF contains white cells and a high protein content but no organisms. This is a multisystem disease and the symptoms and investigations are explained best by a diagnosis of **systemic lupus erythematosus** (SLE). SLE is an autoimmune condition which is about nine times more common in women than men, and is especially common in Afro-caribbeans and Asians. It varies in severity from a mild illness causing a rash or joint pains to a life-threatening multisystem illness. In the brain, SLE causes a small-vessel vasculitis and can present with depression, a schizophrenia-like psychosis, fits, chorea and focal cerebral/spinal cord infarction. Lumbar puncture usually shows a raised leukocyte count and protein level. A Coombs-positive haemolytic anaemia may occur. Leukopenia and thrombocytopenia are common. Glomerulonephritis is another common manifestation of lupus and may present with microscopic haematuria/proteinuria, nephrotic syndrome or renal failure. Arthritis commonly affects the proximal interphalangeal and metacarpophalangeal joints and wrists, usually as arthralgia without any deformity.

> **!** **DIFFERENTIAL DIAGNOSIS OF HEADACHES/PSYCHIATRIC FEATURES/FITS**
>
> - Meningitis/encephalitis
> - 'Recreational' drug abuse (e.g. cocaine)
> - Cerebral tumour
> - Acute alcohol withdrawal (delirium tremens)
> - Hypertensive encephalopathy

This patient needs urgent antihypertensive treatment to lower her blood pressure and anticonvulsant treatment. Blood should be sent for anti-DNA antibodies (present in SLE) and complement C3 and C4 levels (depressed in SLE). A renal biopsy will provide histological evidence of lupus. As soon as active infection has been excluded, treatment should be started with intravenous steroids and cytotoxic agents such as cyclophosphamide. Plasma exchange may be added in severe cases.

> **KEY POINTS**
>
> - SLE is particularly common in young Afro-caribbean women.
> - SLE may present with predominantly neurological or psychiatric features.
> - A low white-cell count or low platelets is often a suggestive feature of SLE.

An 85-year-old man is admitted to hospital because of recurrent falls. These have occurred around eight times over the last three months. He says that the falls have occurred in the morning on most occasions but have occasionally occurred in the afternoon. He does not think that he has lost consciousness although he does remember a sensation of dizziness with the falls. On each occasion he has felt back to normal 5–10 min afterwards. On two or three occasions he has hurt his knees on falling and on one occasion he hit his head. He says that the falls have not been associated with any chest pain or palpitations. He lives alone and there have been no witnesses of any of the falls.

He smokes five cigarettes a day; he does not drink. He has an occasional cough with some white sputum but he cannot remember whether he was coughing at the time of any of the falls. He was diagnosed as having hypertension at a routine check up four years ago and has been on treatment with a diuretic, bendrofluazide, and an α-blocker, doxazosin, for this. The blood pressure has been checked in the surgery on three or four occasions and has been well controlled. He was found to have a high fasting blood sugar six months before and had been advised on a diabetic diet. There is no relevant family history. He worked as a gardener until he retired at the age of 68 years.

On examination he looks well. His pulse is 90/min and irregular. The blood pressure was 134/84. The heart sounds are normal and there is nothing abnormal to find on examination of the respiratory system or gastrointestinal system. There are no significant hypertensive changes in the fundi. In the nervous system, there is a little loss of sensation to light touch in the toes but no other abnormalities.
The ECG is shown in Fig. 53.1.

INVESTIGATIONS

		Normal
Haemoglobin	13.8 g/dl	13.7–17.7 g/dl
Mean corpuscular volume (MCV)	86 fl	80.5–99.7 fl
White cell count	6.9×10^9/l	$3.9–10.6 \times 10^9$/l
Platelet count	288×10^9/l	$150–440 \times 10^9$/l
Sodium	139 mmol/l	135–145 mmol/l
Potassium	4.3 mmol/l	3.5–5.0 mmol/l
Urea	3.9 mmol/l	2.5–6.7 mmol/l
Creatinine	66 μmol/l	70–120 μmol/l
Glucose	6.2 mmol/l	4.0–6.0 mmol/l (fasting)

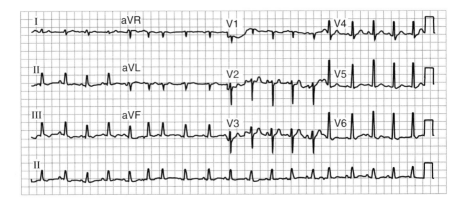

Figure 53.1

QUESTION

- What are the most likely diagnoses?

148

ANSWER 53

There are a number of possibilities to explain falls in the elderly. Some more information in the history about the circumstances of these falls would be helpful. On further enquiry, it emerges that the falls are most likely to occur when he gets up from bed first thing in the morning. The afternoon events have occurred on getting up from a chair after his post-lunch doze. These circumstances suggest a possible diagnosis of **postural hypotension**. This was verified by measurements of standing and lying blood pressure. These results confirmed a marked postural drop with blood pressure decreasing from 134/84 to 102/66. This is likely to be caused by the antihypertensive treatment especially the alpha-blocker which causes vasodilatation. Another possible candidate for a cause of the postural hypotension is the diabetes which could be associated with autonomic neuropathy. In this case the diabetes is not known to have been present for long and there is evidence of only very mild peripheral sensory neuropathy. Diabetic autonomic neuropathy is usually associated with quite severe peripheral sensory with or without motor neuropathy.

The ECG shows evidence of sino-atrial node disease or sick sinus syndrome. Clinically, it is easily mistaken for atrial fibrillation because of the irregular rhythm and the variation in strength of beats. The ECG shows a P-wave with each QRS complex although the P-waves change in shape and timing. It may be associated with episodes of bradycardia and/or tachycardia which could cause falls. This might be investigated further with a 24-hour ambulatory recording of the ECG.

Coughing bouts can cause falls through cough syncope. The positive intrathoracic pressure during coughing limits venous return to the heart. The cough is usually quite marked and he might be expected to remember this since he gives a good account of the falls otherwise. Syncope can occur in association with micturition. Neck movements with vertebrobasilar disease, poor eyesight and problems with balance are other common causes of falls in the elderly. A neurological cause, such as transient ischaemic episodes and epilepsy, is less likely with the lack of prior symptoms and the swift recovery with clear consciousness and no neurological signs.

Another diagnosis which should be remembered in older people who fall is a subdural haematoma. Symptoms may fluctuate and this might be considered and ruled out with a computed tomography (CT) scan of the brain.

The doxazosin should be stopped and another antihypertensive agent started if necessary. This might be a beta-blocker, long-acting calcium antagonist or angiotensin converting-enzyme (ACE) inhibitor although all these can cause postural drops in blood pressure. His symptoms all disappeared on withdrawal of the doxazosin. The blood pressure rose to 154/88 lying and 146/84 standing indicating no significant postural hypotension with reasonable blood-pressure control.

KEY POINTS

- Falls in the elderly are a symptom in need of a diagnosis.
- Postural hypotension is a common side effect of diuretics, vasodilators or other anti-hypertensive therapy. Lying and standing blood pressures should be done if this is suspected.

CASE 54

A 55-year-old man presented to his GP with the results of a routine medical screening undertaken by all employees at his company. He has a family history of ischaemic heart disease in that his father developed angina at the age of 62 years. He is a non-smoker who drinks around 38 units of alcohol a week. He takes little exercise, playing gentle tennis once a fortnight. He is 6 ft tall and weighs 94kg.

INVESTIGATIONS

		Normal
Haemoglobin	13.1 g/dl	(13.7–17.7 g/dl)
Mean corpuscular volume (MCV)	80 fl	(80.5–99.7 fl)
White cell count	6.4×10^9/l	$(3.9–10.6 \times 10^9$/l)
Platelet count	223×10^9/l	$(150–440 \times 10^9$/l)
Erythrocyte sedimentation rate	22 mm	(<10 mm)
Sodium	138 mmol/l	(135–145 mmol/l)
Potassium	3.9 mmol/l	(3.5–5.0 mmol/l)
Urea	4.6 mmol/l	(2.5–6.7 mmol/l)
Creatinine	84 μmol/l	(70–120 μmol/l)
Calcium	2.34 mmol/l	(2.12–2.65 mmol/l)
Phosphate	1.06 mmol/l	(0.8–1.45 mmol/l)
Alkaline phosphatase	84 IU/l	(30–300 IU/l)
Alanine aminotransferase	36 IU/l	(5–35 IU/l)
Gamma glutamyl transpeptidase	68 IU/l	(11–51 IU/l)
Thyroid-stimulating hormone	1.2 mU/l	(<6.0 mU/l)
Cholesterol	5.9 mmol/l	(<5.5 mmol/l)
Fasting glucose	5.2 mmol/l	(4.0–6.0 mmol/l)
Urine	no protein, blood, sugar	
Faeces	positive for blood on biochemical testing	
Electrocardiogram	non-specific T-wave flattening in V5 and V6	

QUESTIONS

- What further investigations are appropriate?
- What abnormalities are present?

ANSWER 54

The most important immediate finding is the **blood in the stool** on routine screening. He requires further investigation of the bowels by repeat occult blood testing and endoscopy of the upper and lower gastrointestinal tract.

There are a number of other features that need attention. He is overweight and does not take enough exercise. The cholesterol level is a little higher than desirable and he has non-specific changes on the ECG which would need further investigation if there was any history of angina or if this developed when he increased his regular exercise. Weight reduction and increased exercise would be likely to reduce his cholesterol level. His alcohol consumption is too high and this may well account for the slightly high gamma-glutamyl transpeptidase result. Alcohol consumption should be reduced below the recommended limit of 28 units per week and the liver-function tests repeated after a period. In the light of the possible bowel abnormality, a liver ultrasound would be appropriate to exclude metastatic disease.

Blood in the faeces, identified visibly or by biochemical testing, requires further investigation. Visible red blood is derived from the lower bowel unless bleeding from the stomach or duodenum is massive. It can come from local lesions around the rectum, such as haemorrhoids or fissures. However, it may be the only sign of a carcinoma of the large bowel. Blood from the upper part of the gastrointestinal tract, such as oesophageal lesions, peptic ulcers or carcinoma of the stomach, is altered by digestion as it passes through the gastrointestinal tract.

No bowel symptoms are reported but this might be questioned further. The haemoglobin and the MCV are at the lower end of the normal range which may suggest that he has been losing more blood. This could be investigated further by measuring the ferritin level to check on the iron stores. In this case, colonoscopy showed a small adenocarcinoma in the descending colon. There was no evidence of any spread. The colonic carcinoma was suitable for resection and would be expected to carry a good prognosis having been found early and completely resected.

✎ KEY POINTS

- The finding of blood loss requires thorough investigation of the gastrointestinal tract.
- Prognosis of carcinoma of the colon depends on the histological grade of malignancy and the degree of spread (Dukes' classification).
- Colorectal cancer causes 18 000 deaths each year in England & Wales; screening for occult blood has been recommended although there is a high incidence of positive results without significant underlying disease other than haemorrhoids, and it is not generally recommended in the UK.

A 33-year-old man presents to his GP complaining of a painless lump on the right side of his neck. This has been present for about two months and seems to be enlarging. He has had no recent throat infections. He has been feeling generally unwell and has lost about 5 kg in weight. The patient has also developed drenching night sweats. He has had no significant past medical history. He is an accountant, married with three children. He neither smokes nor drinks alcohol and is not taking any regular medication.

On examination, his temperature is 37.8°C. There is a smooth, firm 3 × 4 cm palpable mass in the right supraclavicular fossa. There are also lymph nodes 1–2cm in diameter, palpable in both axillae and inguinal areas. His oropharynx appears normal. His pulse rate is 100/min regular and blood pressure 112/66. Examination of his cardiovascular and respiratory systems is normal. On abdominal examination, there is a mass palpable 3 cm below the left costal margin. The mass is dull to percussion and it is impossible to palpate its upper edge. Neurological examination is normal.

INVESTIGATIONS

		Normal
Haemoglobin	12.6 g/dl	(13.3–17.7g/dl)
Mean cell volume	87 fl	(80–99 fl)
White cell count	12.2 × 10⁹/l	(3.9–10.6 × 10⁹/l)
Platelets	321 × 10⁹/l	(150–440 × 10⁹/l)
Erythrocyte sedimentation rate	74 mm/h	(<10 mm/h)
Sodium	138 mmol/l	(135–145 mmol/l)
Potassium	4.2 mmol/l	(3.5–5.0 mmol/l)
Urea	5.2 mmol/l	(2.5–6.7 mmol/l)
Creatinine	114 μmol/l	(70–120 μmol/l)
Calcium	2.44 mmol/l	(2.12–2.65 mmol/l)
Phosphate	1.1 mmol/l	(0.8–1.45 mmol/l)
Total protein	65 g/l	(60–80g/l)
Albumin	41 g/l	(35–50g/l)
Bilirubin	16 μmol/l	(3–17 μmol/l)
Alanine transaminase	22 IU/l	(5–35 IU/l)
Alkaline phosphatase	228 IU/l	(30–300 IU/l)
Urinalysis	no protein; no blood	

QUESTIONS

- What is the likely diagnosis?
- How would you investigate and manage this patient?

ANSWER 55

Transient small nodes in the neck or groin are common benign findings. However, a 3 × 4 cm mass of nodes for two months is undoubtedly abnormal. The swelling in the abdomen has the characteristics of a spleen. Lymphadenopathy, splenomegaly and constitutional symptoms add up to a likely diagnosis of **lymphoma** or chronic leukaemia. Lymph nodes are normally barely palpable, if at all. The character of enlarged lymph nodes is very important. In acute infections the nodes are tender and the overlying skin may be red. Carcinomatous nodes are usually very hard, fixed and irregular. The nodes of chronic leukaemias and lymphomas are non-tender, firm and rubbery. The distribution of enlarged lymph nodes may be diagnostic. Repeated minor trauma and infection may cause enlargement of the locally draining lymph nodes. Enlargement of the left supraclavicular nodes may be due to metastatic spread from bronchial and nasopharyngeal carcinomas or from gastric carcinomas (Virchow's node). However, when there is generalized lymphadenopathy with or without splenomegaly, a systemic illness is most likely. The typical systemic symptoms of lymphoma are malaise, fever, night sweats, pruritus, weight loss, anorexia and fatigue.

! MAJOR DIFFERENTIAL DIAGNOSIS OF LYMPHOMA

- Infections – infectious mononucleosis or 'glandular fever' (caused by Epstein–Barr virus infection), toxoplasmosis, cytomegalovirus infection, tuberculosis, brucellosis and syphilis.
- Inflammatory conditions – systemic lupus erythematosus, rheumatoid arthritis and sarcoidosis.
- Lymphomas or chronic lymphocytic leukaemia.

The most likely clinical diagnosis in this man is lymphoma. The patient should be referred to a local oncology unit. He should have a lymph-node biopsy to reach a histological diagnosis, and a computed tomography (CT) scan of thorax and abdomen and bone marrow to stage the disease. CT scanning is a non-invasive and effective method of imaging retroperitoneal, iliac and mesenteric nodes. Prior to its advent, patients were often subjected to a 'staging laparotomy'. The patient will require treatment with radiotherapy and chemotherapy. Radiotherapy alone is reserved for patients with limited disease, but this patient has widespread disease. He should be given allopurinol prior to starting chemotherapy to prevent massive production of uric acid as a consequence of tumour lysis.

✎ KEY POINTS

- The character and distribution of lymph nodes is helpful in reaching a diagnosis.
- Lymphadenopathy affecting two separate groups suggests lymphoma or a systemic infection.

A 63-year-old woman has been told that she has become rather yellow and when she arrives at the surgery she is found to be jaundiced. The jaundice was noticed when her niece came to stay with her. She has been unwell for around two years with chronic fatigue. Recently she has been anorexic but is unclear whether she has lost any weight. Her other complaints are of itching for two to three months but she has not noticed any skin rash. In answer to direct questions she says that her mouth and eyes have felt dry.

There has been no disturbance of her bowels or urine although she thinks that her urine has been rather 'strong' lately. She is 12 years postmenopausal. In her previous medical history, she has had hypothyroidism for which she has been taking thyroxine replacement in a dose of 150 μg daily for ten years. There is a family history of thyroid disease. She does not smoke and drinks less than five units of alcohol each week. She has never drunk more than this regularly. She has taken occasional paracetamol for headaches but has been on no regular medication other than thyroxine.

On examination, her sclerae are yellow and she has xanthelasmata around the eyes. There are excoriated marks from her scratching over her back and her upper arms. The pulse is 74/min and regular, blood pressure is 128/76. No abnormalities are found in the cardiovascular or respiratory system. In the abdomen, the liver is not palpable but the spleen is felt 2 cm under the left costal margin.

INVESTIGATIONS

		Normal
Sodium	142 mmol/l	135–145 mmol/l
Potassium	4.2 mmol/l	3.5–5.0 mmol/l
Urea	5.6 mmol/l	2.5–6.7 mmol/l
Creatinine	84 μmol/l	70–120 μmol/l
Calcium	2.24 mmol/l	2.12–2.65 mmol/l
Phosphate	1.09 mmol/l	0.8–1.45 mmol/l
Total bilirubin	124 μmol/l	3–17 μmol/l
Alkaline phosphatase	764 IU/l	30–300 IU/l
Alanine aminotransferase	65 IU/l	5–35 IU/l
Gamma-glutamyl transpeptidase	788 IU/l	11–51 IU/l
Thyroid stimulating hormone	1.3 mU/l	0.3–6.0 mU/l
Cholesterol	7.8 mmol/l	<5.5 mmol/l
Fasting glucose	4.7 mmol/l	4.0–6.0 mmol/l
Antinuclear antibody	+	
Antimitochondrial antibody	+++	
Thyroid antibodies	++	

QUESTIONS

- What is your interpretation of these findings?
- What is the likely diagnosis and how might this be confirmed?

ANSWER 56

The liver function tests show a predominantly obstructive picture with high alkaline phosphatase while cellular enzymes are only slightly raised. The symptoms and investigations are characteristic of **primary biliary cirrhosis**, an uncommon condition found mainly in middle-aged women. In the liver there is chronic inflammation around the small bile ducts in the portal tracts. Hypercholesterolaemia, xanthelasmata and xanthomata are common. The dry eyes and dry mouth may occur as part of an associated sicca syndrome. Itching occurs because of raised levels of bile salts and can be helped by the use of a binding agent such as cholestyramine which interferes with their reabsorption.

Hypothyroidism might explain some of her symptoms but the normal thyroid-stimulating hormone (TSH) level shows that this is adequately controlled by the current dose of 150 μg thyroxine. The thyroid antibodies reflect the autoimmune thyroid disease which is associated with other autoantibody-linked conditions such as primary biliary cirrhosis. The presence of antimitochondrial antibodies in the blood is typical of primary biliary cirrhosis. These antibodies are found in 95 per cent of cases.

The diagnosis is confirmed by a liver biopsy. This should only be carried out after an ultrasound confirms that there is no obstruction of larger bile ducts. This will help to rule out other causes of obstructive jaundice although the clinical picture described here is typical of primary biliary cirrhosis. No treatment is known to affect the clinical course of this condition.

✑ KEY POINTS

- The pattern of liver enzyme abnormalities usually reflects either an obstructive or hepatocellular pattern.
- Symptoms such as itching have a wide differential diagnosis. Dealing with the underlying cause, wherever possible, is preferable to symptomatic treatment.

A 22-year-old woman complains of tiredness and mild abdominal discomfort with gradual increase in frequency of bowel movements from once a day in her teens to two to three times daily. The discomfort is variable and usually in the centre of the abdomen. She says that the bowel movements can be difficult to flush away on occasions but this is not a consistent problem. Her tiredness has been present for four months or more. She is a non-smoker and drinks rarely. She has been a vegetarian for five years but eats dairy foods and fish regularly and her appetite has been normal. She thinks that her grandmother, who lived in Ireland, had some bowel problems but she died three years ago, aged 68.

On examination, she is 5 ft 4 in tall and weighs 49 kg. She looks a little pale and thin. Examination of her abdomen showed no abnormalities and there are no other significant abnormalities to find in any other system.

▲ BLOOD TESTS

		Normal
Haemoglobin	10.7 g/dl	11.7–15.7 g/dl
Mean corpuscular volume (MCV)	98 fl	80.8–100.0 fl
White cell count	6.5 × 10⁹/l	3.5–11.0 × 10⁹/l
Platelet count	247 × 10⁹/l	150–440 × 10⁹/l
Red cell folate	44 μg/l	>160 μg/l
Vitamin B12	280 ng/l	176–925 ng/l
Thyroid stimulating hormone	3.5 mU/l	0.3–6.0 mU/l
Free thyroxine	12.9 pmol/l	9.0–22.0 pmol/l

The blood film is reported as a dimorphic film with remnants of nuclear material (Howell–Jolly bodies) in some of the red blood cells.

QUESTIONS

- How do you interpret these findings?
- What is the likely diagnosis and how might this be confirmed?

ANSWER 57

The most likely diagnosis is malabsorption from **coeliac disease.** The report of a dimorphic blood film means that there are both small and large cells. This suggests that the anaemia is caused by a combination of the folate deficiency indicated by the red cell folate and by iron deficiency. The Howell–Jolly bodies are dark blue regular inclusions in the red cells which are typically found in the blood of patients after splenectomy or are associated with the splenic atrophy which is characteristic of coeliac disease. In coeliac disease, there is a sensitivity to dietary gluten, a water-insoluble protein found in many cereals. The proximal small bowel is the main site involved with loss of villi and an inflammatory infiltrate causing reduced absorption.
The MCV is at the upper limit of normal.

! CAUSES OF MACROCYTOSIS IN THE BLOOD FILM

- Folate deficiency
- Vitamin B_{12} deficiency
- Hypothyroidism
- Abnormal liver function

Coeliac disease is made more likely by a possible positive family history and the origin from Ireland where coeliac disease is four times as common as in the rest of the UK.

Diagnosis can be confirmed by endoscopy at which a biopsy can be taken from the distal duodenum. Typically this will show complete villus atrophy. Antigliadin antibodies are usually positive. The treatment is a gluten-free diet with a repeat of the biopsy some months later to show improvement in the height of the villi in the small bowel. In some cases, temporary treatment with steroids may be needed to help recovery. Another common cause of failure to recover the villus architecture is poor compliance to the difficult dietary constraints.

⚲ KEY POINTS

- Howell–Jolly bodies are characteristic of hyposplenism.
- Coeliac disease can present at any age with non-specific symptoms.
- Typical features of fat malabsorption may not be evident if the patient eats a diet with little or no fat intake.

CASE 58

A 30-year-old man has a history of a persistent cough. He has consulted his GP on three occasions over six months and two courses of antibiotics have had no effect. The cough is most troublesome when going out in to cold air and on jogging. It has also woken him up from his sleep on several occasions. The only medical history he can remember is that he had recurrent episodes of bronchitis as a child between the ages of 5 and 6 years. He has never smoked and takes no medication. He has two brothers, one of whom has mild seasonal rhinitis. His parents are alive and well.

His GP organized a chest X-ray which was reported as normal. He arranged respiratory function tests at the local hospital and the results are shown below. He asked the patient to record his peak expiratory flow at home morning and evening for two weeks. The results are plotted in Fig 58.1.

On examination, no abnormalities were found in the nose, pharynx, cardiovascular or respiratory systems.

RESPIRATORY FUNCTION TEST

	Actual	Predicted
FEV$_1$ (l)	4.0	3.8–4.4
FVC (l)	5.2	4.8–5.6
FER (FEV$_1$/FVC) (%)	77	75–80
PEF (L/min)	475	480–580

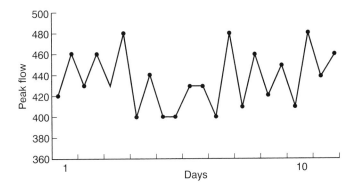

Figure 58.1 Peak flow recording

QUESTIONS

- What is your interpretation of these findings?
- What do you think is the likely diagnosis and what would be appropriate treatment?

ANSWER 58

The peak flow pattern shows a degree of diurnal variation. This does not reach the diagnostic criteria for **asthma** but it is suspicious. The mean daily variation in peak flow from the recordings is 36 l/min and the mean evening peak flow is 453 l/min giving a mean diurnal variation of 8 per cent. There is a small diurnal variation in normals and a variation of > 15 per cent is diagnostic of asthma. In this patient the label of 'bronchitis' as a child was probably asthma. The family history of an atopic condition (hayfever in a brother), the triggering of the cough by exercise and cold air also suggests bronchial hyperresponsiveness typical of asthma.

Patients with a chronic persistent cough of unexplained cause should have a chest X-ray. When the X-ray is clear the cough is likely to be produced by one of three main causes. Around half of such cases have asthma or will go on to develop asthma over the next few years. Half the rest have rhinitis or sinusitis with a post-nasal drip. In around 20 per cent the cough is related to gastro-oesophageal reflux. A small number of cases will be caused by otherwise unsuspected problems such as foreign bodies, bronchial 'adenoma', sarcoidosis or fibrosing alveolitis. Cough is a common side effect in patients treated with angiotensin converting-enzyme (ACE) inhibitors.

In this patient the diagnosis of asthma was confirmed with an exercise test which was associated with a 25 per cent drop in peak flow. Alternatives would have been another non-specific challenge such as methacholine or histamine or a therapeutic trial of inhaled steroids. After the exercise test, an inhaled steroid was given and the cough settled after one week. The inhaled steroid was discontinued after two weeks and replaced by a β_2-agonist to use before exercise. However, the cough recurred with more evident wheeze and shortness of breath and treatment was changed back to an inhaled steroid with a β_2-agonist as needed. In some cases, the persistent dry cough associated with asthma may require more vigorous treatment than this. Inhaled steroids for a month or more or even a two-week course of oral steroids may be needed to relieve the cough. The successful management of dry cough relies on establishing the correct diagnosis and treating it vigorously.

ᕍ KEY POINTS

- The three commonest causes of persistent dry cough with a normal chest X-ray are asthma (50 per cent), sinusitis and postnasal drip (25 per cent) and reflux oesophagitis (20 per cent).
- Asthma may present as a cough (cough variant asthma) with little or no airflow obstruction initially, although this develops later.

CASE 59

A 54-year-old woman presents to the casualty department complaining of breathlessness and generalized muscular weakness. She has become increasingly weak over the past six months, and now has difficulty getting out of a chair. Her breathing has become increasingly laboured over the past few days. She also complains of a headache, lack of appetite and nausea. She was diagnosed with Sjögren's syndrome two years previously. She has no other significant past medical history. She is a non-smoker and drinks 5 units of alcohol per week. She is on no medication.

On examination her pulse is 92/min, blood pressure 130/84, jugular venous pressure not raised, heart sounds normal with no peripheral oedema. Her respiratory rate is 30/min, but her breath sounds are normal. Abdominal examination is normal. Muscle power is generally reduced. Tone, reflexes, coordination and sensation are normal.

INVESTIGATIONS

		Normal
Haemoglobin	13.1 g/dl	(11.7–15.7 g/dl)
White cell count	10.2×10^9/l	($3.5–11.0 \times 10^9$/l)
Platelets	350×10^9/l	($150–440 \times 10^9$/l)
Sodium	135 mmol/l	(135–145 mmol/l)
Potassium	1.9 mmol/l	(3.5–5.0 mmol/l)
Bicarbonate	8 mmol/l	(24–30 mmol/l)
Chloride	115 mmol/l	(95–105 mmol/l)
Urea	6.4 mmol/l	(2.5–6.7 mmol/l)
Creatinine	90 μmol/l	(70–120 μmol/l)
Arterial blood gases (on air)		
pH	7.23	(7.38–7.44)
pCO_2	3.1 kPa	(4.7–6.0 kPa)
pO_2	13.2 kPa	(12.0–14.5 kPa)
Urinary pH	7.0	
ECG	sinus tachycardia	
Chest X-ray	normal	

QUESTIONS

- What metabolic abnormality is present?
- How would you manage this patient?

ANSWER 59

This woman has a hyperchloraemic hypokalaemic metabolic acidosis. The severe hypokalaemia is causing her profound muscle weakness. The low pH and bicarbonate indicate the presence of acidosis, and the low pCO_2 is due to stimulation of the respiratory centre by the acidosis causing compensatory hyperventilation. Metabolic acidosis causes non-specific symptoms, namely breathlessness, headache, anorexia and nausea. The causes of a metabolic acidosis are classified according to the presence of an increased or normal anion gap. The anion gap is calculated from the biochemical results by the equation $Na^+ + K^+ - [Cl^- + HCO_3^-]$. Normal values for the anion gap are between 10 and 18 mmol/l.

! CAUSES OF METABOLIC ACIDOSIS

Normal anion gap
- Gastrointestinal losses of bicarbonate
- Ureteroenterostomy
- Proximal renal tubular acidosis
- Distal renal tubular acidosis

Increased anion gap
- Diabetic ketoacidosis
- Lactic acidosis
- Alcoholic ketoacidosis
- Uraemia
- Toxins – salicylates, methanol, ethylene glycol, paraldehyde

This patient has a normal anion gap (14 mmol/l) and the presence of a urine pH > 5.4 (i.e. not appropriately acidified) in the presence of acidosis suggests **distal renal tubular acidosis** (RTA). In distal RTA patients who are not acidotic, the inability to acidify the urine normally can be demonstrated by giving an ammonium chloride load. Distal RTA may be idiopathic or may be associated with diseases that specifically damage the distal tubule such as Sjögren's disease or amphotericin B nephrotoxicity.

Proximal RTA is commoner in children and is due to diseases which affect the proximal tubule's ability to reabsorb filtered bicarbonate. Loss of bicarbonate may cause systemic acidosis, but the ability to form an acid urine when acidosis becomes severe is retained; the response to ammonium chloride loading is therefore normal.

This patient must initially have her hypokalaemia corrected with intravenous potassium. Correction of the acidosis without adequate potassium replacement may cause life-threatening hypokalaemia by redistributing extracellular potassium into cells. Long-term treatment requires 2–3 mmol/kg oral sodium bicarbonate per day.

✎ KEY POINTS

- Calculation of the anion gap is an essential first step in the evaluation of a patient with metabolic acidosis.
- Patients with distal and proximal renal tubular acidosis are distinguished by the inability of the former to acidify their urine appropriately.

A 43-year-old woman presents to her GP complaining of generalized weakness. She has noticed difficulty holding her head up, especially in the evenings. She has problems finishing a meal because of difficulty chewing. Her husband and friends have noticed that her voice has become quieter. She has lost about 3 kg of weight in the past six months. The woman has had no significant previous medical illnesses. She lives with her husband and three children. She is a non-smoker and drinks about 15 units of alcohol per week. She is taking no regular medication.

On examination, she looks well and examination of cardiovascular, respiratory and abdominal systems is normal. Power in all muscle groups is grossly normal but decreases after testing a movement repetitively. Tone, coordination, reflexes and sensation are normal. Bilateral ptosis is present and is exacerbated by prolonged upward gaze. Pupillary reflexes, eye movements and fundoscopy are normal.

QUESTIONS

- What is the diagnosis?
- What are the major differential diagnoses?
- How would you investigate and manage this patient?

ANSWER 60

This woman's generalized weakness is due to **myasthenia gravis**. Myasthenia gravis is due to the presence of acetylcholine receptor antibodies causing impaired neuro-muscular transmission. It characteristically affects the external ocular, bulbar, neck and shoulder girdle muscles. Weakness is worse after repetitive movements which cause acetylcholine depletion from the presynaptic terminals. The onset is usually gradual. Ptosis of the upper lids is often associated with diplopia due to weakness of the exter-nal ocular muscles. Speech may become soft when the patient is tired. Symptoms are usually worse in the evenings and better in the mornings. Permanent paralysis even-tually develops in some muscle groups. In severe cases respiratory weakness occurs.

! DIFFERENTIAL DIAGNOSES OF GENERALIZED MUSCLE WEAKNESS

- Motor neurone disease – suggested clinically by muscle fasciculation and later by marked muscle weakness.
- Muscular dystrophies – selective muscular weakness occurs in specific dis-eases, e.g. facioscapulohumeral dystrophy. There is usually a family history.
- Dystrophia myotonica – this causes ptosis, wasting of the masseter, temporal and sternomastoid muscles and distal muscular atrophy. There is a character-istic facial appearance with frontal baldness, expressionless facies and sunken cheeks. There may be gonadal atrophy and mental retardation. There is usual-ly a family history. The EMG is diagnostic.
- Polymyositis – this may have an acute or chronic onset. A skin rash and joint pains are common. The creatine kinase level is raised and a muscle biopsy is diagnostic.
- Miscellaneous myopathies: thyrotoxic, hypothyroid, Cushing's, alcoholic.
- Non-metastatic associations of malignancy, e.g. the Eaton–Lambert syndrome associated with carcinoma of the bronchus.

This patient should be investigated by a neurologist. EMG will demonstrate fatiguabil-ity in response to repetitive supramaximal stimulation. Intravenous injection of edro-phonium (Tensilon) will increase muscular power for a few minutes. Blood should be assayed for acetylcholine receptor antibodies (present in 90 per cent). A computed tomography (CT) thorax should be performed to detect the presence of a thymoma. Corticosteroids are the drugs of first choice. Anticholinesterase drugs greatly improve muscle power but have many side effects. Thymectomy should be considered. It is most effective within five years of diagnosis and when there is no thymoma.

⚲ KEY POINTS

- Myasthenia gravis is a cause of abnormal muscular fatiguability.
- In its initial stages it affects certain characteristic muscle groups.

A 64-year-old man goes to his GP because he has become increasingly overweight. He has gained 8 kg in weight over the past six months. He has noticed that he is constantly hungry. He has found that he is bruising easily. He finds it difficult to get up from his armchair or to climb his stairs. He feels depressed and finds himself waking early in the mornings. He has had no previous physical or psychiatric illnesses. He is a retired miner and lives with his wife. He smokes 30 cigarettes per day and drinks 15 units of alcohol per week.

On examination, he is overweight particularly in the abdominal region. There are purple stretch marks on his abdomen and thighs. His pulse is 76/min, regular and blood pressure 168/104. There is peripheral oedema. Otherwise examination of his heart, respiratory and abdominal systems is normal. His neurological examination is otherwise normal, apart from some weakness in shoulder abduction and hip flexion.

INVESTIGATIONS

		Normal
Haemoglobin	13.2 g/dl	(13.3–17.7g/dl)
Mean cell volume	87 fl	(80–99 fl)
White cell count	5.2×10^9/l	($3.9–10.6 \times 10^9$/l)
Platelets	237×10^9/l	($150–440 \times 10^9$/l)
Sodium	138 mmol/l	(135–145 mmol/l)
Potassium	3.3 mmol/l	(3.5–5.0 mmol/l)
Urea	6.2 mmol/l	(2.5–6.7 mmol/l)
Creatinine	113 µmol/l	(70–120 µmol/l)
Albumin	38 g/l	(35–50 g/l)
Glucose	8.3 mmol/l	(4.0–6.0 mmol/l)
Bilirubin	16 µmol/l	(3–17 µmol/l)
Alanine transaminase	24 IU/l	(5–35 IU/l)
Alkaline phosphatase	92 IU/l	(30–300 IU/l)
Gamma-glutamyl transpeptidase	43 IU/l	(11–51 IU/l)
Urinalysis	– protein; – blood; + + glucose	

QUESTIONS

- What is the likely diagnosis?
- How would you investigate and manage this patient?

ANSWER 61

The symptoms and signs of proximal myopathy, striae and truncal obesity suggest **Cushing's syndrome**. The hyperglycaemia and hypokalaemia would fit this diagnosis. In addition psychiatric disturbances, typically depression, may occur in Cushing's syndrome. This patient's primary presenting complaint is rapid onset obesity. The principal causes of obesity are:

- Genetic
- Environmental – excessive food intake, lack of exercise
- Hormonal – hypothyroidism, Cushing's syndrome, polycystic ovaries and hyperprolactinaemia
- Alcohol-induced pseudo-Cushing's syndrome

! CAUSES OF CUSHING'S SYNDROME

- Adrenocorticotrophic hormone (ACTH) secretion by a basophil adenoma of the anterior pituitary gland (Cushing's disease).
- Ectopic ACTH secretion e.g. from a bronchial carcinoma, often causing a massive release of cortisol and a severe and rapid onset of symptoms.
- Primary adenoma/carcinoma of the adrenal cortex (suppressed ACTH).
- Iatrogenic – corticosteroid treatment.

This patient should be investigated by an endocrinologist. The first point is to establish that this man has abnormal cortisol secretion. There should be loss of the normal diurnal rhythm with an elevated midnight cortisol level or increased urinary conjugated cortisol excretion. A dexamethasone suppression test would normally suppress cortisol excretion. It is then important to exclude common causes of abnormal cortisol excretion such as stress/depression or alcohol abuse. Measurement of ACTH levels distinguishes between adrenal (low ACTH) and pituitary/ectopic causes (high ACTH). This patient drinks alcohol moderately and has a normal gamma-glutamyl transpeptidase. His depression seems to be a consequence of his cortisol excess rather than a cause, as he has no psychiatric history.

His ACTH level is elevated. Bronchial carcinoma is a possibility as he is a heavy smoker and the onset of his Cushing's syndrome has been rapid. However his chest X-ray is normal. In this man a MRI scan (T1-weighted coronal image) through the pituitary shows a hypointense microadenoma (Fig. 61.1, arrow). This can be treated with surgery or radiotherapy.

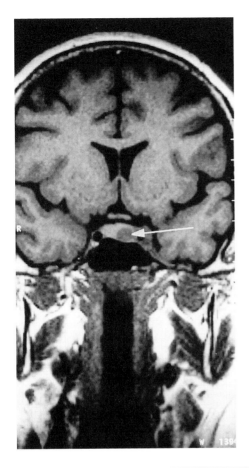

Figure 61.1 MRI scan through pituitary

- Patients with rapid-onset obesity should have endocrine causes excluded.
- Patients with severe and rapid-onset Cushing's disease often have ectopic ACTH secretion or cortisol-secreting adrenal tumours.

CASE 62

A 35-year-old man is admitted to the casualty department having been found unconscious in his bathroom by his wife on her return from work in the evening. He has suffered from insulin-dependent diabetes mellitus for 18 years and his diabetic control is poor. He has never had an episode of diabetic ketoacidosis but has had recurrent hypoglycaemic episodes. Over the past few weeks he has developed cellulitis on his right foot and received two courses of oral antibiotics. He has recently complained to his wife of fatigue, polyuria, polydipsia and anorexia. Two years previously he suffered a myocardial infarction. He has had bilateral laser treatment for proliferative diabetic retinopathy. The man is unemployed and lives with his wife. He smokes 15 cigarettes per week and drinks 20 units of alcohol per week. His treatment is twice-daily insulin.

On examination he is clinically dehydrated with reduced skin turgor and poor capillary return. His breath smells sweet. His pulse is low volume, regular and 116/min. His blood pressure is 92/70 lying, 72/50 sitting up. His respiratory rate is 30/min with deep sighing breaths. Otherwise, examination of his respiratory and abdominal systems is normal. He has an infected foot ulcer on his left foot. He is rousable only to painful stimuli. There is no focal neurology. Fundoscopy shows bilateral scars as a result of laser therapy.

INVESTIGATIONS

		Normal
Haemoglobin	14.2 g/dl	(11.7–15.7 g/dl
White cell count	14.3 × 10⁹/l	(3.5–11.0 × 10⁹/l)
Platelets	321 × 10⁹/l	(150–440 × 10⁹/l)
Sodium	140 mmol/l	(135–145 mmol/l)
Potassium	5.8 mmol/l	(3.5–5.0 mmol/l)
Chloride	105 mmol/l	(95–105 mmol/l)
Urea	12.3 mmol/l	(2.5–6.7 mmol/l)
Creatinine	136 μmol/l	(70–120 μmol/l)
Bicarbonate	10 mmol/l	(24–30 mmol/l)
Glucose	34.4 mmol/l	(4.0–6.0 mmol/l)
Urinalysis	++ protein; ++ ketones; +++ glucose	
Blood gases on air		
	pH 7.28	(7.38–7.44)
	pCO_2 2.8 kPa	(4.7–6.0 kPa)
	pO_2 12.2 kPa	(12.0–14.5 kPa)

QUESTIONS

- What is the cause for this man's coma?
- How would you manage this patient?

ANSWER 62

This man has signs of dehydration and the high urea with a normal creatinine is consistent with this. The blood glucose level is raised and he is acidotic. This patient has **hyperglycaemic ketoacidotic coma**. The key clinical features on examination are dehydration, hyperventilation and ketosis. A persistently high sugar level induced by his infected foot ulcer causes heavy glycosuria triggering an osmotic diuresis. This leads to hypovolaemia and reduced renal blood flow causing prerenal uraemia. The extracellular hyperosmolality causes severe cellular dehydration, and loss of water from his brain cells is the cause of his coma. Decreased insulin activity with intracellular glucose deficiency stimulates lipolysis and the production of ketoacids. He has a high anion gap metabolic acidosis due to accumulation of ketoacids (acetoacetate and 3-hydroxybutyrate). The anion gap is calculated from the equation $Na^+ + K^+ - [Cl^- + HCO_3^-]$ and is normally 10–18 mmol/l and in this case is 31 mmol/l. Ketones cause a characteristically sickly sweet smell on the breath of patients with diabetic ketoacidosis (about 20 per cent of the population cannot smell the ketones). The metabolic acidosis stimulates the respiratory centre leading to an increase in the rate and depth of respiration (Kussmaul breathing). In older diabetic patients there is often evidence of infection precipitating these metabolic abnormalities (e.g. bronchopneumonia, infected foot ulcer).

The differential diagnosis of coma in diabetics includes non-ketotic hyperglycaemic coma, particularly in elderly diabetics, lactic acidosis especially in patients on metformin, profound hypoglycaemia, and non-metabolic causes for coma, e.g. cerebrovascular attacks and drug overdose. Salicylate poisoning may cause hyperglycaemia, hyperventilation and coma but the metabolic picture is usually one of a dominant respiratory alkalosis and mild metabolic acidosis.

The aims of management are to correct the massive fluid and electrolyte losses, hyperglycaemia and metabolic acidosis. Rapid fluid replacement with intravenous normal saline and potassium supplements should be started. In patients with cardiac or renal disease, a central venous pressure (CVP) line is mandatory. Regular monitoring of plasma potassium is essential as it may fall very rapidly as glucose enters cells (ECG monitoring is needed). Insulin therapy is usually given by intravenous infusion with monitoring of blood glucose levels. A nasogastric tube is essential to prevent aspiration of gastric contents, and a bladder catheter to measure urine production. Antibiotics and local wound care should be given to treat this man's foot ulcer. In the longer term it is important that this patient and his wife are educated about his diabetes and that he has regular access to diabetes services.

🔍 KEY POINTS

- Dehydration, tachypnoea and ketosis are the key clinical signs of diabetic ketoacidosis.
- Twenty per cent of the population (and therefore doctors) cannot smell ketones.

CASE 63

A 45-year-old woman is admitted to hospital with pneumonia. She has had three episodes of cough, fever and purulent sputum over the last six months. One of these was associated with right-sided pleuritic chest pain. These have been treated at home by her GP. In addition she has a five-year history of difficulty with swallowing. Initially this was mild but it has become progressively worse. She says that food seems to stick in the low retrosternal area. This applies to all types of solid food. She has lost 5 kg in weight over the last two months. Sometimes the difficulty with swallowing seems to improve during a meal. Recently she has had trouble with regurgitation and vomiting of recognizable food.

Three years ago her GP arranged for an outpatient upper gastrointestinal endoscopy which was normal. She was reassured but the problem has increased in severity. There is no other relevant medical history or family history. She lived in the north-west coast of the United States for four years up until ten years ago. She works as a shop assistant. She has never smoked and drinks less than 5 units of alcohol each week. There has been no disturbance of micturition. She has always tended to be constipated and this has been a little worse recently.

On examination, she looks thin. In the respiratory system there are some crackles at the right base. There are no abnormalities to find in the abdomen.

Her chest X-ray is shown in Fig. 63.1.

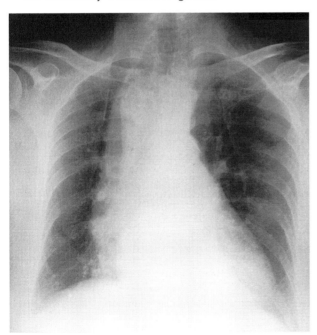

Figure 63.1 Chest X-ray. (Reproduced with the kind permission of the authors from *Radiology for the MRCP* by Curtis and Whitehouse, published by Arnold in 1998.)

QUESTION

- What is the likely diagnosis and how would you establish this?

ANSWER 63

The likely diagnosis is **achalasia of the cardia**, a primary neurological disturbance of the nerve plexuses at the lower end of the oesophagus. The X-ray shows a dilated fluid-filled oesophagus with no visible gastric air bubble. Endoscopy may be normal in the early stages as in this case. The oesophagus has now dilated and there has been spill-over of stagnant food into the lungs giving her the episodes of repeated respiratory infections. Such aspiration is most likely to affect the right lower lobe because of the more vertical right main bronchus although the result of aspiration at night may depend on the position of the patient. The dysphagia is often variable early on. It tends to be present for all foods indicating a motility problem and there may initially be some relief from the mechanical load as the oesophagus fills. Dysphagia for bulky, solid foods first usually indicates an obstructive lesion.

The diagnosis can be made at this stage by a barium swallow showing the dilated oesophagus. Earlier it may require careful cine-radiology with a bolus of food impregnated with barium or oesophageal motility studies using a catheter fitted with a number of pressure sensors to detect the abnormal motility of the oesophageal muscle.

A similar condition can be produced by the protozoan parasite *Trypanosoma cruzi* (Chagas' disease) but this is limited to South and Central America and would not be relevant to her stay in the north-west United States.

Other common causes of dysphagia might be benign oesophageal strictures from acid reflux, malignant strictures, external compression or an oesophageal pouch. Achalasia may be managed by muscle relaxants when mild but often requires treatment to disrupt the lower oesophageal muscle by dilatation or surgery.

KEY POINTS

- The subjective site of blockage in dysphagia may not reflect accurately the level of the obstruction.
- Persistent dysphagia without explanation needs investigation by barium swallow or endoscopy.

CASE 64

A 74-year-old woman has a ten-year history of intermittent lower abdominal pain. The pain has been colicky in nature and associated with a feeling of distension in the left iliac fossa. It is generally relieved by passing flatus or faeces. She tends to be constipated and passes small pieces of faeces. Four years previously she passed some blood and had a barium enema performed. This is shown in Fig. 64.1.

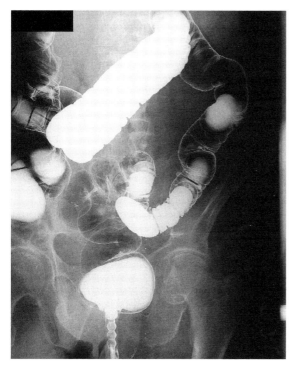

Figure 64.1 Barium enema

Over the last week her pain has worsened and now she has continuous pain in the left iliac fossa and feels generally unwell. Her appetite has been poor over this same time. She has not had her bowels open over the last two days. In her previous medical history she had a hysterectomy for fibroids 20 years ago. There is a family history of ischaemic heart disease and diabetes mellitus. She lives alone and does her own cooking and shopping.

On examination, she has a temperature of 38.5°C and is tender with a vague impression of a mass in the left iliac fossa. There is no guarding or rebound tenderness and the bowel sounds are normal. Her pulse is 90/min and blood pressure is 104/68. There are no abnormalities to find in the respiratory system.

INVESTIGATIONS

		Normal
Haemoglobin	11.8 g/dl	11.7–15.7 g/dl
Mean corpuscular volume (MCV)	85 fl	80.8–100.0 fl
White cell count	15.6 × 10⁹/l	3.5–11.0 × 10⁹/l
Platelet count	235 × 10⁹/l	150–440 × 10⁹/l

QUESTIONS

- What is the likely diagnosis?
- What should be the initial management?

ANSWER 64

The barium enema from four years ago shows evidence of **diverticular disease** with outpouchings of the mucosa in the sigmoid colon. This would be consistent with the long-standing history of abdominal pain of colonic type and tendency to constipation. The recent problems with increased pain, tenderness, fever, raised white count and a mass in the left iliac fossa would be compatible with an acute exacerbation of her diverticular disease. There is no evidence of peritonitis which would signal a possible perforation of one of the diverticula.

The differential diagnosis, with the suggestion of a mass and change in bowel habit, would be carcinoma of the colon and Crohn's disease. In the absence of evidence of perforation with leak of bowel contents into the peritoneum (no peritonitis) or obstruction (normal bowel sounds, no general distension), treatment should be based on the presumptive diagnosis of acute diverticular disease with further investigation, if appropriate, after the acute changes have settled.

An ultrasound examination of the abdomen would help to delineate the mass and suggest whether there was evidence of local abscess formation. Treatment should include broad-spectrum antibiotics, intravenous fluids and rest. Further investigations are indicated, including electrolytes, urea and creatinine, liver-function tests, blood cultures and, in view of the family history, blood sugar and colonoscopy should be considered. Repeated severe episodes, bleeding or obstruction might necessitate surgery.

✎ KEY POINTS

- Diverticular disease is a common finding in the elderly.
- Diverticular disease is a common condition; its presence can distract the unwary doctor from pursuing a co-incident condition.

A 45-year-old man consults his GP because of loss of libido. He has been feeling generally less well for two years but has not sought medical help before. He has had some pains in the knees particularly after any exercise. He has felt more lethargic and short of energy. At the end of the day, he has noticed a little swelling of the ankles.

In the family history, his parents are both alive and well. His paternal uncle died of heart failure and cirrhosis in his fifties. His grandfather had diabetes and liver disease and died at 50 years of age.

He works as a bricklayer, smokes 20 cigarettes daily and drinks 15 units of alcohol a week. His weight is steady and there is no disturbance of bowels or micturition. He has no cough and no chest pain or palpitations.

On examination, he has some generalized skin pigmentation. The liver is palpable 3 cm under the right costal margin. A third heart sound is audible and the jugular venous pressure is raised 3 cm. The blood pressure is 126/82 and the heart rate 80/min. There is minimal ankle oedema. There is some testicular atrophy and loss of secondary sex hair.

BLOOD TESTS

		Normal
Haemoglobin	16.1 g/dl	(13.7–17.7 g/dl)
Mean corpuscular volume (MCV)	88 fl	(80.5–99.7 fl)
White cell count	6.9×10^9/l	(3.9–10.6×10^9/l)
Platelet count	286×10^9/l	(150–440×10^9/l)
Sodium	137 mmol/l	(135–145 mmol/l)
Potassium	4.3 mmol/l	3.5–5.0 mmol/l
Urea	4.3 mmol/l	(2.5–6.7 mmol/l)
Creatinine	77 μmol/l	(70–120 μmol/l)
Calcium	2.28 mmol/l	(2.12–2.65 mmol/l)
Phosphate	1.09 mmol/l	(0.8–1.45 mmol/l)
Alkaline phosphatase	124 IU/l	(30–300 IU/l)
Alanine aminotransferase	56 IU/l	(5–35 IU/l)
Gamma-glutamyl transpeptidase	76 IU/l	(11–51 IU/l)
Thyroid-stimulating hormone	1.7 mU/l	(0.3–6.0 mU/l)
Fasting glucose	8.2 mmol/l	(4.0–6.0 mmol/l)
Serum iron	62 μmol/l	(14–31 μmol/l)
Total iron-binding capacity	68 μmol/l	(45–70 μmol/l)

QUESTIONS

- What is your interpretation of these findings?
- What is the likely diagnosis?

ANSWER 65

The likely diagnosis is **haemochromatosis**. The abnormal blood tests are mildly raised liver-function tests, glucose is raised and there is a high iron with normal iron-binding capacity. In this condition, the ferritin level measuring iron stores would be very high. Haemochromatosis is an autosomal recessive condition in which too much iron is absorbed from the bowel. The excess iron accumulates in a number of organs and this excess of iron would be seen in a liver biopsy. Accumulation occurs also in the testes, joints, heart and pancreas. This would explain many of the other features here such as arthralgia, glucose intolerance, decreased libido, feminization and early heart failure. One in 250 of a northern European population have the homozygous genetic abnormality but not all are affected clinically. Men are affected more often than women (9 : 1) and presentation is most often between 40 and 60 years.

Loss of libido may be associated with psychological problems or be related to underlying illness or drug therapy. It requires a careful and sensitive history and clinical examination.

Ferritin is the best blood test to assess iron stores. They can also be assessed directly by staining a bone-marrow sample for iron. Ferritin is an acute-phase protein and is raised non-specifically in acute illnesses. If a serum iron level is low, then the level of the iron-binding capacity should be measured. If both iron and total iron-binding capacity are low, chronic disease is the likely cause of anaemia. In iron deficiency, the serum iron is low but iron-binding capacity is high in an attempt to capture as much iron as possible.

Haemochromatosis could explain the medical history in his grandfather and paternal uncle. If the diagnosis is confirmed other male family members should be investigated to rule out haemochromatosis. The commonest genetic mutation has been identified and genetic studies can help in diagnosis. Treatment is by venesection to remove iron. This is monitored by measurements of haemoglobin and ferritin (for iron stores).

Treatment may require venesection at two-weekly intervals for one or two years to get the iron levels down.

The liver biopsy would show excess iron accumulation and liver cell damage. There is a risk of hepatocellular carcinoma in haemochromatosis.

Hereditary haemochromatosis is an autosomal recessive condition and the gene, *HFE*, and two mutations have been identified. The severity is determined by an interaction between genotype and modifying factors such as gender, iron and alcohol intake.

🔍 KEY POINTS

- Serum iron, iron-binding capacity and ferritin can all be used to assess iron stores but their limitations must be appreciated.
- Regular venesections can control iron stores in haemochromatosis.

CASE 66

A 69-year-old widower smoked 40 cigarettes a day for over 50 years but then gave up six months ago when his wife died of carcinoma of the lung. He has had a cough with daily sputum production for the last 30 years and has become increasingly short of breath. His sputum is either white or yellow in colour. He has put on weight recently and now weighs 110 kg. He says that his ankles have been swollen recently and his exercise tolerance has dropped to about 100 yards on the flat and to half a flight of stairs before he has to stop. He worked as a bricklayer for 38 years and has become frustrated by his inability to do what he used to do. It has become too much effort to walk to his local public house and he is having difficulty getting his shopping from the local store.

His GP has given him a bronchodilator metered-dose inhaler which produced a slight improvement in his symptoms. A course of 30 mg prednisolone daily for 5 days was given also but he developed indigestion. Nevertheless he persevered with the tablets and noticed no change during the course or any deterioration when he stopped them.

On examination, he is overweight. He appears to be centrally cyanosed and has bilateral ankle oedema. His jugular venous pressure is raised 3 cm. He has a large anteroposterior chest diameter. There are some early inspiratory crackles at the lung bases and an expiratory wheeze.

His chest X-ray is shown in Fig. 66.1. Lung-function tests were performed.

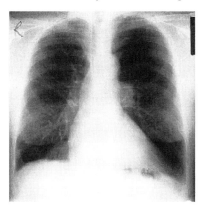

Figure 66.1

RESPIRATORY FUNCTION TESTS

	Actual	Predicted
FEV₁ (l)	0.45	3.5–4.3
FVC (l)	1.25	4.6–5.4
FER (FEV₁/FVC) (%)	36	72–80
PEF (l/min)	90	440–540

QUESTIONS

- What is the likely diagnosis?
- What management is appropriate?

ANSWER 66

The most likely diagnosis is **chronic obstructive pulmonary disease** (COPD). The physical signs and chest X-ray indicate overinflation. The early inspiratory crackles are typical of COPD.

The bronchodilator response should be pursued looking at the effect of β_2-agonists and anticholinergic agents. Theophylline may sometimes be useful as a third-line therapy but has more side effects.

Ideally, the steroid trial should be for three weeks (five days is certainly too short). It should be monitored with respiratory-function tests but the lack of any subjective improvement makes it unlikely that there will be a response. More often the problem is to differentiate the subjective euphoric effect, sometimes produced by steroids, from a true effect on the airways backed up by any changes in the physiological tests or exercise tolerance.

He is cyanosed and has signs of right-sided heart failure (cor pulmonale). Blood gases should be checked to see if he might be a candidate for long-term home-oxygen therapy (known to improve survival if paO_2 in the steady-state breathing air remains < 7.2 kPa). Gentle diuresis might help the oedema although oxygen would be a better approach if he is sufficiently hypoxic. Annual influenza vaccination should be recommended and *streptococcus pneumoniae* vaccination should be considered. Antibiotics might be kept at home for infective exacerbations.

Exercise tolerance will be reduced by his obesity and by lack of muscle use. A weight-reducing diet should be started. If he has the motivation to continue exercising, then a pulmonary rehabilitation programme has been shown to increase exercise tolerance by 10–20 per cent and to improve quality of life. Other more dramatic interventions such as lung-reduction surgery or transplantation might be considered in a younger patient.

COPD is often regarded as a condition where treatment has little to offer. However, a vigorous approach tailored to the need of the individual patient can provide a worthwhile benefit.

🔑 KEY POINTS

- In COPD β_2-agonists and anticholinergic agents produce similar effects or a greater response from anticholinergics. The combination may be helpful. In contrast, in asthma β_2-agonists produce a greater effect.
- Assessment for home oxygen should be made in a stable state on optimal other therapy.

CASE 67

A 76-year-old lady is referred by her GP to a nephrologist for investigation of hypertension and renal impairment. She has been known to be hypertensive for eight years. Five years prior to this referral she had an inferior myocardial infarction. She also suffers from pain in both legs on walking more than 100 yards. Blood tests done by the GP two months ago show a creatinine of 204 mmol/l. There is no family history of hypertension or renal disease. She has smoked 20 cigarettes for 50 years and drinks 10 units of alcohol per week. She is widowed, but has two children who live nearby.

On examination, her pulse rate is 92/min irregular, blood pressure 180/90, jugular venous pressure not raised, heart sounds normal. A left carotid bruit is audible. No pedal pulses are palpable. Examination of the chest and abdomen is normal apart from a bruit audible over the umbilicus.

The nephrologist organizes the following investigations:

INVESTIGATIONS

		Normal
Haemoglobin	13.1 g/dl	(11.7–15.7 g/dl)
Mean cell volume	82 fl	(80–99 fl)
White cell count	10.3×10^9/l	(3.5–11.0×10^9/l)
Platelets	187×10^9/l	(150–440×10^9/l)
Sodium	137 mmol/l	(135–145 mmol/l)
Potassium	3.6 mmol/l	(3.5–5.0 mmol/l)
Urea	10.1 mmol/l	(2.5–6.7 mmol/l)
Creatinine	212 μmol/l	(70–120 μmol/l)
Glucose	4.6 mmol/l	(4.0–6.0 mmol/l)
Albumin	38 g/l	(35–50g/l)
Cholesterol	8.4 mmol/l	(3.9–7.8 mmol/l)
Triglyceride	2.3 mmol/l	(0.55–1.90 mmol/l)
Urinalysis	no protein; no blood	
Renal ultrasound	Right kidney 11.5 cm; left kidney 7.2 cm	

QUESTIONS

- What is the likely cause for this patient's hypertension and renal impairment?
- How would you further investigate and manage this patient?

ANSWER 67

This woman presents with hypertension and renal impairment shown by the raised creatinine. She is a smoker and has evidence of generalized atherosclerosis manifested by a previous myocardial infarction, a carotid bruit and bilateral claudication with loss of peripheral pulses. The asymmetrical axial length of the kidneys in a patient who is an arteriopath is highly suggestive of **renovascular disease**. Her small left kidney implies that she has a left renal artery occlusion, and the raised serum creatinine suggests that the right renal artery has a significant stenosis which is causing a reduction in function of the right kidney. The abdominal bruit is likely to originate from one of the renal arteries. Renovascular disease is being recognized increasingly as a cause of renal failure. Patients with atheromatous renal arterial disease are usually arteriopaths and have a high mortality from strokes and myocardial infarctions.

This patient had a renal angiogram performed (Fig. 67.1). Alternative non-invasive techniques for imaging the renal arteries include Doppler ultrasound, spiral computed tomography (CT) and MRI angiography. Angiography in this case confirms a right proximal renal artery stenosis (arrow) and a left renal artery occlusion (the artery is not visualized). The patient could be considered for angioplasty of the right renal artery stenosis. The role of angioplasty is controversial but its main role appears to be to prevent progression to total occlusion of the artery (which would lead this patient to require dialysis). Angioplasty has unpredictable effects on improving blood-pressure control or serum creatinine levels. This patient should have her blood pressure controlled with antihypertensive agents. Angiotensin-converting enzyme inhibitors should be avoided in patients with renal arterial disease as they can precipitate acute renal failure. This is because the glomerular filtration rate in kidneys supplied by a stenosed artery is maintained by angiotensin II-mediated constriction of the efferent glomerular arteriole. She should also be advised to stop smoking and be given a statin to lower her serum cholesterol level which is raised.

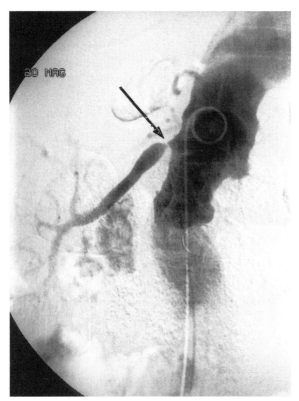

Figure 67.1

- Renal arterial disease is a common cause of renal failure in the elderly population.
- Clues to the presence of renovascular disease include generalized vascular disease, a heavy smoking history, hypertension and asymmetrically-sized kidneys on renal ultrasound.

A 55-year-old woman goes to her GP complaining of painful fingers and toes. Her fingers have caused her pain for many years but have become worse recently. She has noticed that exposing her hands to the cold causes her fingers to turn blue and then red, numb and painful. Recently she has developed a discharge of a white chalky material from the tip of her left forefinger. She has suffered from long-standing heartburn but now has difficulty swallowing unless she sits absolutely upright. She is also breathless on walking up hills or climbing stairs, but is not breathless on lying flat. There is no significant past medical history. She is an accountant and neither smokes tobacco nor drinks alcohol. She is on no medication.

On examination, the skin appears very tight on the backs of her hands and is difficult to pick up. There is a small ulcer on the left forefinger discharging white calcific material. There is radial furrowing of the skin around her mouth and her mouth appears small. Telangiectasiae are present on her face. Her pulse is 76/min regular and blood pressure 130/85. Her heart sounds are soft with no added sounds. Chest expansion is reduced bilaterally and on auscultation diffuse bilateral fine late inspiratory crackles are audible. Examination of the abdominal and neurological systems is normal.

INVESTIGATIONS

		Normal
Haemoglobin	12.2 g/dl	(11.7–15.7 g/dl)
White cell count	6.2×10^9/l	(3.5–11.0×10^9/l)
Platelets	178×10^9/l	(150–440×10^9/l)
Erythrocyte sedimentation rate	8 mm/h	(<10 mm/h)
Sodium	136 mmol/l	(135–145 mmol/l)
Potassium	4.4 mmol/l	(3.5–5.0 mmol/l)
Urea	5.4 mmol/l	(2.5–6.7 mmol/l)
Creatinine	113 μmol/l	(70–120 μmol/l)
Glucose	4.3 mmol/l	(4.0–6.0 mmol/l)
Urinalysis	no protein; no blood	

QUESTIONS

- What is the diagnosis?
- How would you investigate and manage this patient?

ANSWER 68

This woman gives a long history of Raynaud's phenomenon affecting her fingers and toes associated more recently with cutaneous ulceration and calcinosis. Calcinosis is easily mistaken for gouty tophi discharging uric acid crystals. She has the **CREST variant of systemic sclerosis (SSc)**. Systemic sclerosis has two major categories – diffuse cutaneous SSc and limited cutaneous SSc. Patients with limited cutaneous SSc usually have skin sclerosis restricted to their hands and face and may suffer from the CREST syndrome. CREST is an acronym for the combination of **C**alcinosis, **R**aynaud's disease, o**E**sophageal involvement, **S**clerodactyly and **T**elangiectasia. Her dysphagia is due to atrophy of the muscle coat of the lower oesophagus causing loss of neuromuscular coordination, acid reflux and stricture formation. Characteristically in the CREST variant, the disease progresses very slowly and is only rarely associated with renal disease. Its major complication is severe pulmonary hypertension secondary to pulmonary vascular disease and diffuse interstitial pulmonary fibrosis. This lady has the reduced chest expansion and fine late inspiratory crackles of pulmonary fibrosis. Her heart sounds are soft due to a pericardial effusion. In contrast, in diffuse cutaneous SSc, more skin on the trunk and limbs is involved and there is a higher incidence of significant renal, lung and cardiac disease.

Raynaud's disease may be idiopathic or associated with other factors

! FACTORS ASSOCIATED WITH RAYNAUD'S DISEASE

- Systemic lupus erythematosus
- Mixed connective-tissue disease
- Cervical rib/thoracic outlet syndromes
- β-blockers
- Cryoglobulinaemia
- Long-term use of vibrating tools

This lady should be referred to a rheumatologist for further investigation. Blood should be sent to the clinical immunology laboratory for detection of antinuclear factor, anticentromere antibody (usually present in CREST syndrome) and anti-Scl 70 antibody (associated with increased risk of pulmonary fibrosis). A barium swallow should be performed to assess her lower oesophagus. Respiratory function tests and a high-resolution computed tomography (CT) thorax will delineate pulmonary involvement, with an echocardiogram to look at the right ventricle and pulmonary artery pressures. CT thorax (Fig. 68.1a) in this patient demonstrates a pericardial effusion (short arrow) and dilated oesophagus (long arrow) and in the lung fields (Fig. 68.1b) shows pulmonary fibrosis (arrow).

The patient should be advised to keep her fingers and toes warm. Infected ulcers should be treated with antibiotics. Nifedipine causes peripheral vasodilatation and improves Raynaud's disease. Metoclopramide and ranitidine help the oesophageal motility disorder and reflux oesophagitis.

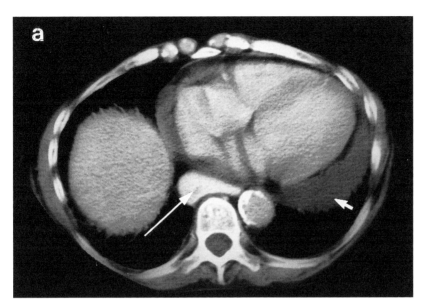

Figure 68.1a CT thorax

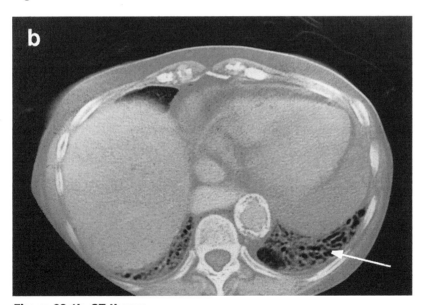

Figure 68.1b CT thorax

🔍 KEY POINTS

- Raynaud's disease may be idiopathic or part of a multisystem disease.
- Patients with limited cutaneous SSc often have CREST syndrome and may develop pulmonary fibrosis late (> 10 years) after initial presentation.
- Patients with diffuse cutaneous SSc are at high risk of cardiac, pulmonary and renal involvement within five years of presentation.

A 63-year-old man presents to his GP complaining that over the past three months he has developed severe generalized itching. This is particularly severe after a hot bath. He has also noticed frequent headaches, dizziness and tinnitus. He has been hypertensive for 10 years. He smokes 35 cigarettes a day and drinks about 25 units of alcohol per week. He takes bendrofluazide for his hypertension. He works as a chef, is divorced and lives alone.

On examination his face looks plethoric. There are no signs of chronic liver disease and no lymphadenopathy. His pulse is 84/min regular and blood pressure 162/104. Examination of his heart and respiratory system is normal. His spleen is palpable 4 cm below the left costal margin. Neurological examination is normal.

INVESTIGATIONS

		Normal
Haemoglobin	18.6 g/dl	(13.3–17.7g/dl)
Mean cell volume	88 fl	(80–99 fl)
White cell count	14.2×10^9/l	$(3.9–10.6 \times 10^9$/l)
Platelets	411×10^9/l	$(150–440 \times 10^9$/l)
Sodium	137 mmol/l	(135–145 mmol/l)
Potassium	4.6 mmol/l	(3.5–5.0 mmol/l)
Urea	6.4 mmol/l	(2.5–6.7 mmol/l)
Creatinine	84 μmol/l	(70–120 μmol/l
Bilirubin	12 μmol/l	(3–17 μmol/l)
Alanine transaminase	24 IU/l	(5–35 IU/l)
Alkaline phosphatase	68 IU/l	(30–300 IU/l)
Urinalysis	no protein; no blood	

QUESTIONS

- What is the likely diagnosis?
- What are the major causes of generalized itching?
- How would you investigate and manage this patient?

ANSWER 69

This patient has **polycythaemia rubra vera**. This is due to abnormal proliferation of red cell precursors derived from a single haematopoietic progenitor cell with the capacity for differentiation down red cell, white cell and platelet lines. As a result, there is an increase in haemoglobin, white cell count and platelet level. Patients may present with a thrombotic event or with symptoms due to increased blood viscosity such as headaches, tinnitus and blurred vision. There is an increased bleeding tendency. Splenomegaly is common. Severe pruritus is characteristic and is particularly related to warmth occurring on getting into a warm bed or bath.

! CONDITIONS ASSOCIATED WITH GENERALIZED PRURITUS

- Obstructive jaundice due to bile salt retention
- Iron deficiency
- Lymphoma
- Carcinoma, especially bronchial
- Chronic renal failure, partially due to phosphate retention

This patient should be referred to a haematology unit for investigation. It is important to exclude relative polycythaemia due to dehydration from diuretic and alcohol use. In polycythaemia rubra vera, the red cell mass will be raised but normal in relative polycythaemia. The following causes of secondary polycythaemia must be excluded:

- Chronic lung disease with hypoxia
- Cyanotic congenital heart disease
- Renal cysts, tumours, renal transplants
- Hepatoma, cerebellar haemangioblastoma, uterine fibroids
- Cushing's disease

The erythropoietin level is low in polycythaemia rubra vera and high in secondary polycythaemia. Pulse oximetry or arterial blood gases should be performed to exclude hypoxia. The leukocyte alkaline phosphatase level is also raised in polycythaemia rubra vera.

The patient should be venesected until the haematocrit is within the normal range. A variety of agents can be used to keep the haematocrit down: ^{32}P, hydroxyurea and busulphan. The disease may transform into acute leukaemia or myelosclerosis.

✎ KEY POINTS

- Severe generalized pruritus is a characteristic symptom of polycythaemia rubra vera.

A 40-year-old man complains of abdominal pain which has been present intermittently for six months. The pain is in the lower part of the abdomen where it varies between the right iliac fossa and the central suprapubic area. He eats a good diet but has lost 5 kg in weight over this period. There have been mild disturbances of bowel habit ranging from diarrhoea to constipation. He has had problems with peri-anal pain and was found to have an anal fissure two months previously. There is no relationship between the timing or intensity of the pain and any particular food. Over the last three weeks he has felt feverish on occasions.

He is a smoker of 10 cigarettes daily and drinks 10 units of alcohol weekly. He is on no medication. He has no previous relevant medical history or family history.

On examination, the pulse rate is 74/min, blood pressure 124/80. In the abdomen there is a little tenderness in the right iliac fossa and in the same area an ill-defined mass of around 6 cm diameter is palpable. The bowel sounds are normal. There are some thick skin tags at the anal margin and a chronic anal fissure. Examination of cardiovascular and respiratory systems is normal and there are no other skin lesions.

BLOOD TESTS

		Normal
Haemoglobin	12.2 g/dl	13.3–17.7 g/dl
Mean corpuscular volume (MCV)	88 fl	80.5–99.7 fl
White cell count	$10.6 \times 10^9/l$	$3.9–10.6 \times 10^9/l$
Platelet count	$245 \times 10^9/l$	$150–440 \times 10^9/l$
Erythrocyte sedimentation rate	74 mm	<10 mm in 1 h

QUESTIONS

- How do you interpret these findings?
- What is the most likely diagnosis and how could this be confirmed?

ANSWER 70

The most likely diagnosis is **Crohn's disease** (regional enteritis). The long history of abdominal discomfort with the ill-defined abdominal mass and the peri-anal problems are very suggestive of Crohn's disease. Loops of bowel often adhere to each other and the peritoneum to form an inflammatory mass. Peri-anal lesions, often fleshy skin tags, occur frequently. The mild anaemia and the raised erythrocyte sedimentation rate (ESR) would also fit with this diagnosis. The aetiology of Crohn's disease is unknown, infective and toxic causes have been suggested. Environmental factors probably modulate a genetic predisposition indicated by human leukocyte antigen (HLA) linkages.

In acute illnesses of this sort *Yersinia enterocolitica* ileitis would be a possible differential and *Mycobacterium tuberculosis* should be remembered in chronic cases. Carcinoma of the caecum can be difficult to diagnose without skilful colonoscopy.

The diagnostic procedure should be small bowel radiology which would be expected to show focal ulcers and may show strictures and fistulae. Histological confirmation might be produced by colonoscopy or by resection of a limited area of affected bowel. Crohn's disease may affect any part of the gastrointestinal tract and has a tendency to produce strictures and fistulae.

In this case, the disease seemed to be localized to the terminal part of the ileum. It was controlled by the introduction of prednisolone with relief of pain, raising of the haemoglobin and reduction in the ESR. He should be seen by a dietitian with a view to nutritional supplements. Sulphasalazine or mesalazine helps when there is colonic involvement and azathioprine may be used as a steroid-sparing agent.

⚲ KEY POINTS

- Peri-anal lesions (skin tags and fissures) are common findings in Crohn's disease.
- Crohn's disease can affect any part of the gastrointestinal tract from the mouth to the anal margin.

A 28-year-old woman presents to her GP complaining that for the past nine months she has been experiencing episodes consisting of severe pounding headaches, sweating, palpitations and intense anxiety lasting for about 20 min. These attacks have been increasing in frequency and now occur on an almost daily basis. They seem to be triggered by bending or laughing. She has not lost weight and her appetite is good. She has had no previous medical illnesses. She is a dental assistant and is married with three children. She is a non-smoker and drinks alcohol occasionally. She is on no medication.

On examination, she looks healthy. Her pulse rate is 72/min regular, and blood pressure 156/94. Fundoscopy shows silver-wiring and arteriovenous nipping. Her examination is otherwise normal. The GP orders investigations.

INVESTIGATIONS

		Normal
Haemoglobin	14.3 g/dl	(11.7–15.7 g/dl)
Mean cell volume	85 fl	(80–99 fl)
White cell count	8.2×10^9/l	$(3.5–11.0 \times 10^9$/l)
Platelets	365×10^9/l	$(150–440 \times 10^9$/l)
Sodium	138 mmol/l	(135–145 mmol/l)
Potassium	4.2 mmol/l	(3.5–5.0 mmol/l)
Bicarbonate	27 mmol/l	(24–30 mmol/l)
Urea	6.7 mmol/l	(2.5–6.7 mmol/l)
Creatinine	104 μmol/l	(70–120 μmol/l)
Glucose	5.6 mmol/l	(4.0–6.0 mmol/l)
Albumin	39 g/l	(35–50 g/l)
Urinalysis	no protein; no blood	
ECG	sinus rhythm, borderline left-ventricular hypertrophy	

QUESTIONS

- What is the likely diagnosis?
- How would you investigate and manage this patient?

ANSWER 71

This lady has features suggestive of a **phaeochromocytoma**. The symptoms and signs are due to very high levels of catecholamines and include paroxysmal hypertension accompanied by anxiety, sweating, headache and either facial pallor or flushing. The attacks may be triggered by physical pressure on the tumour, e.g. bending or tightening a belt, and usually last between 15 and 60 min. The differential diagnosis of the attacks includes anxiety states, thyrotoxicosis, hypoglycaemic attacks, unstable angina, carcinoid syndrome and the delirium tremens of alcohol withdrawal. The hypertension is often persistent rather than paroxysmal. This patient is persistently hypertensive with signs of end-organ damage (left-ventricular hypertrophy and hypertensive retinopathy).

Phaeochromocytomas arise in chromaffin cells of neuroectodermal origin. 90 per cent occur in the adrenal medulla and 10 per cent are extra-adrenal. Ten per cent of adrenal phaechromocytomas are bilateral, and more commonly when they are familial. About 10 per cent of all phaeochromocytomas are malignant.

> **❗ PHAEOCHROMOCYTOMAS AS PART OF OTHER SYNDROMES**
>
> - Multiple endocrine neoplasia type 2 – medullary carcinoma of the thyroid, parathyroid adenoma and multiple neuromata
> - Neurofibromatosis
> - Von Hippel–Lindau disease – renal carcinoma, retinal angiomata and cerebellar haemangioblastoma

This patient should be referred to a hypertension clinic for further investigation. Plasma noradrenaline/adrenaline levels are assayed and 24-hour urinary samples are measured for noradrenaline, adrenaline, dopamine and vanillylmandelic levels. These assays may need to be repeated as hypersecretion of catecholamines may be episodic. Phaeochromocytomas should be imaged with computed tomography (CT) scanning and nuclear medicine scanning.

CT scan (Fig. 71.1) in this patient shows a large right adrenal phaeochromocytoma (arrow). ^{131}I-meta-iodobenzylguanidine (MIBG) is selectively taken up by adrenergic cells. ^{131}I-MIBG scan (Fig. 71.2) in another patient demonstrates a left adrenal phaeochromocytoma on a 24-hour image (arrow). Surgery is the treatment of choice and may cure the hypertension if there have been no irreversible vascular changes. Adequate α- and β-blockade must be established before surgery.

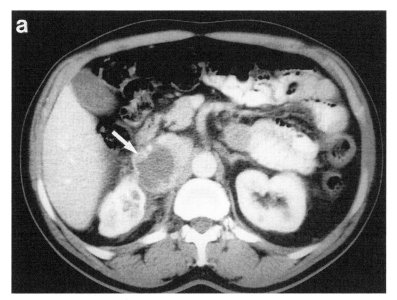

Figure 71.1 CT scan

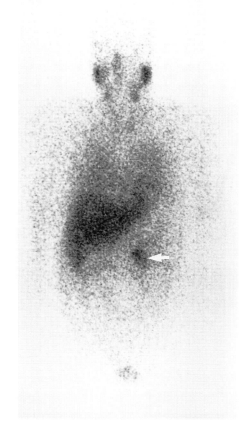

Figure 71.2 ^{131}I-MIBG scan

- Patients presenting with hypertension under the age of 40 years should be investigated for secondary causes of hypertension.
- Common secondary causes of hypertension include chronic renal failure, renal artery stenosis and the oral contraceptive. Rare causes include primary hyper-aldosteronism and coarctation of the aorta.

A 29-year-old man presents with a cough and some mild aches in the hands, wrists and ankles. The symptoms have been present for two months and have increased slightly over that time. Six weeks before he had some soreness of his eyes which resolved in one week.

The cough has been non-productive. He had noticed some skin lesions on the edge of the hairline and around his nostrils. Previously he had been well apart from an appendicectomy at the age of 17 years.

He was born in Trinidad and came to the UK at the age of four years. His two brothers and parents are well. He works as a messenger. On examination of the joints there is no deformity and no evidence of any acute inflammation. In the respiratory and cardiovascular system there are no abnormal findings. In the skin there are some slightly raised areas on the edge of the hairline posteriorly and at the ala nasae. They are a little lighter than the rest of the skin.

The chest X-ray is shown in Fig 72.1.

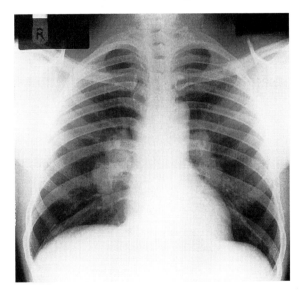

Figure 72.1 Chest X-ray

		Normal
Haemoglobin	13.5 g/dl	(13.0–17.0 g/dl)
Mean corpuscular volume (MCV)	88 fl	(80.5–99.7 fl)
White cell count	8.5×10^9/l	($3.5–11.0 \times 10^9$/l)
Platelet count	264×10^9/l	($150–440 \times 10^9$/l)
Erythrocyte sedimentation rate	34 mm	(<10mm/h)
Sodium	140 mmol/l	(135–145 mmol/l)
Potassium	4.0 mmol/l	(3.5–5.0 mmol/l)
Urea	3.6 mmol/l	(2.5–6.7 mmol/l)
Creatinine	74 μmol/l	(70–120 μmol/l)
Bilirubin	14 μmol/l	(3–17 μmol/l)
Alkaline phosphatase	84 IU/l	(30–300 IU/l)
Alanine aminotransferase	44 IU/l	(5–35 IU/l)
Calcium	2.69 mmol/l	(2.12–2.65 mmol/l)
Phosphate	1.20 mmol/l	(0.8–1.45 mmol/l)

QUESTIONS

- What is the likely diagnosis?
- How might this be confirmed?

ANSWER 72

The likely diagnosis is **sarcoidosis**. The age is typical and sarcoidosis is more common in those of Afro-Caribbean origin. The chest X-ray shows bilateral hilar lymphadenopathy. The blood results show a slightly raised calcium level which is related to vitamin D sensitivity in sarcoidosis where the granulomas hydroxylate 25-hydroxy-cholecalciferol to 1,25-dihydroxycholecalciferol. The erythrocyte sedimentation rate (ESR) is raised and some of the liver enzymes are around the upper limit of normal. The skin lesions at the hairline and the nostrils are typical sites for sarcoid skin problems. The eye trouble six weeks earlier might also have been a manifestation of sarcoidosis which can cause both anterior and posterior uveitis.

An alternative diagnosis which might explain the findings is tuberculosis. Tuberculosis can also cause hypercalcaemia although this is much less common than in sarcoid. Tumours, especially lymphoma, might give this X-ray appearance but would not explain the other findings. The arthralgia (pains with no evidence of acute inflammation or deformity on examination) can occur in sarcoid or tuberculosis but again they are commoner in sarcoid. The ESR is non-specific. Arthralgia without deformity in an Afro-Caribbean man raises the possibility of systemic lupus erythematosus (SLE) but this would be much commoner in women and would not cause bilateral hilar lymphadenopathy

He is likely to have had BCG vaccination at school at around the age of 12 giving a degree of protection against tuberculosis. A tuberculin test should be positive after BCG, strongly positive in most cases of tuberculosis and negative in 80 per cent of cases of sarcoidosis. The serum level of angiotensin-converting enzyme would be raised in over 80 per cent of cases of sarcoidosis but often in tuberculosis also. Histology of affected tissue would confirm the clinical diagnosis. This might be obtained by a skin biopsy of one of the lesions. A bronchial or transbronchial lung biopsy at fibreoptic bronchoscopy would be another means of obtaining diagnostic histology. In patients with a cough and sarcoidosis the bronchial mucosa itself often looks abnormal and biopsy will provide the diagnosis. A gallium scan will show uptake in affected areas in sarcoid, tuberculosis and lymphoma. Sarcoidosis produces a typical appearance with uptake in lacrimal and salivary glands as well as the affected lymph nodes.

Steroid treatment would not be necessary for the hilar lymphadenopathy alone but would be indicated for the hypercalcaemia and possibly for the systemic symptoms.

✎ KEY POINTS

- Sarcoidosis is commoner in Afro-Caribbeans.
- Typical sites for skin lesions are around the nose and the hairline.

A 83-year-old man presents to his GP having developed multiple blisters on his skin and mouth. The blisters have appeared over 2 days. They tend to burst rapidly to leave a large red sore lesion. The patient has lost about 5 kg in weight over the past three months and has a poor appetite.

He has also noticed that his bowel habit has become erratic and that he has developed rectal bleeding. He feels generally unwell. He has previously been fit and had no significant past medical illnesses. He lives alone and neither smokes nor drinks alcohol. He is taking no regular medication.

On examination he looks emaciated and unwell. There are blisters spread over his skin and sores within his mouth. Most of the blisters appear to have burst. His pulse rate is 102/min irregularly irregular and blood pressure 160/78. Examination of his heart and respiratory system is otherwise normal. There is a 6 cm hard nodular liver edge palpable and also a hard mobile mass present in the left iliac fossa. On rectal examination there is some bright red blood mixed with faecal material on the glove.

◤ BLOOD TESTS

		Normal
Haemoglobin	9.2 g/dl	(13.3–17.7g/dl)
White cell count	6.2 × 10⁹/l	(3.9–10.6 × 10⁹/l)
Platelets	236 × 10⁹/l	(150–440 × 10⁹/l)
Mean cell volume	72 fl	(80–99 fl)
Sodium	136 mmol/l	(135–145 mmol/l)
Potassium	3.8 mmol/l	(3.5–5.0 mmol/l)
Urea	5.2 mmol/l	(2.5–6.7 mmol/l)
Creatinine	94 μmol/l	(70–120 μmol/l)
Albumin	32 g/l	(35–50 g/l)
Glucose	4.3 mmol/l	(4.0–6.0 mmol/l)
Bilirubin	16 μmol/l	(3–17 μmol/l)
Alanine transaminase	34 IU/l	(5–35 IU/l)
Alkaline phosphatase	692 IU/l	(30–300 IU/l)
Blood film	hypochromic, microcytic red cells	

QUESTIONS

- What is the diagnosis of the skin disease?
- What is the cause of this condition in this patient?

Answer 73

This patient has **pemphigus vulgaris**. This is a blistering disease where the level of the blister is within the epidermis. The superficial nature of the blister means that the blisters are prone to burst leaving a glistening red base which bleeds easily. The epidermis at the edge of the blister is easily dislodged by sliding pressure (Nikolsky sign). Erosions in the mouth are also common. Associated diseases include carcinoma, lymphoma, thymoma, systemic lupus erythematosus and certain drugs such as penicillamine and captopril.

This elderly man also has hepatomegaly. With the rectal bleeding and microcytic anaemia, it is likely that he has a left-sided colonic neoplasm. The raised alkaline phosphatase suggests secondary metastases in his liver. He needs an ultrasound to image his liver and a colonoscopy to visualize his colon. He should be referred to a surgeon to assess if palliative surgery is appropriate.

Pemphigus is itself life-threatening either due to insensible fluid losses or septicaemia as a result of infection of the exposed blisters. The sore mouth and eroded skin need careful nursing. Treatment is with high doses of corticosteroids and cytotoxic drugs may need to be added.

! Main differential diagnoses of blistering diseases

- Pemphigoid. The level of bullae are deeper (subepidermal) and the blisters are larger and rupture less often than in pemphigus.
- Erythema multiforme. There are target-shaped lesions with central blisters, often with generalized erythema and mucosal ulceration (Stevens–Johnson syndrome). This is often associated with herpes simplex virus infection, certain drugs, e.g. sulphonamides and neoplasms.
- Dermatitis herpetiformis. There are vesicular lesions over the elbows, knees and face. Vesicles are smaller than blisters (< 0.5cm) and often ruptured by itching. This rash is associated with coeliac disease.
- Miscellaneous blistering disorders. Diabetes mellitus, herpes gestationis and familial blistering disorders.

ᖰ Key Points

- Pemphigus is often associated with underlying serious medical conditions.
- Pemphigus may be fatal usually due to septicaemia as a result of superadded infection of blisters and immunosuppressive treatment.

CASE 74

A 71-year-old man complains of general malaise which has been present for three to four weeks. He thinks that he might have lost a few kilogrammes in weight over this time, but does not weigh himself regularly. He says that he has felt limited on exertion by tiredness for a year or so and on three or four occasions when he had tried to do more he had a feeling of tightness across his chest. There is no other medical history of note. He smokes 20 cigarettes per day and drinks around 5 units of alcohol each week. He is not on any medication. On systems review, he says that he has lost his appetite over the last few weeks. His sleep has been disturbed by occasional nocturia and on a few occasions by sweating at night.

There is no relevant family history. He is a retired shopkeeper who normally keeps reasonably fit walking his dog.

On examination, he has a pulse of 70/min, blood pressure of 110/66. The jugular venous pressure is not raised. The apex beat is displaced 2 cm from the midclavicular line. On auscultation of the heart there is an ejection systolic murmur radiating to the carotids and a soft early diastolic murmur audible at the lower left sternal edge. The spleen is palpable 2 cm under the left costal margin. The urine looked clear but routine stick testing showed a trace of blood and on urine microscopy there were some red cells. A chest X-ray was reported as showing a slightly large heart. The electrocardiogram is shown in Fig. 74.1

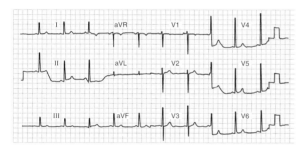

Figure 74.1 ECG

BLOOD TESTS

		Normal
Haemoglobin	10.8 g/dl	(13.3–17.7 g/dl)
Mean corpuscular volume (MCV)	89 fl	(80.5–99.1 fl)
White cell count	11.2×10^9/l	$(3.9–10.6 \times 10^9$/l)
Platelet count	287×10^9/l	$(150–440 \times 10^9$/l)
Erythrocyte sedimentation rate	68 mm in 1 h	(<20 mm in 1 h)

QUESTIONS

• What is the most likely diagnosis?
• What investigations are indicated?

ANSWER 74

This 71-year-old man has the clinical features of aortic stenosis and regurgitation. The murmurs are of mixed aortic valve disease and the ECG shows left ventricular hypertrophy (sum of negative deflection in V1 and positive deflection in V5 or V2 and V6 greater than 35 mm) suggesting that there has been significant pressure overload from aortic stenosis. The findings of mixed aortic valve disease, microscopic haematuria, splenomegaly, malaise and fever (likely from the night sweats) make **infective endocarditis** a likely diagnosis. This would fit with the haematological picture showing a normocytic anaemia, a marginally raised white cell count and a high erythrocyte sedimentation rate (ESR). In the elderly, infective endocarditis may be an insidious illness and should be considered in any patient who has murmurs and fever or any other change in the cardiac signs or symptoms. The other classical findings of splinter haemorrhages, clubbing, Osler's nodes, Janeway lesions and Roth's spots are often absent. Precipitating events such as dental treatment or other sources of bacteraemia may not be evident in the history.

It is difficult to tie all the features into any other single diagnosis. The signs are of aortic valve disease. When there is a fever or other evidence of infection in the presence of valve disease infective endocarditis must always be considered although in practice other unrelated infections are more common. Other infections such as tuberculosis or abscess are possible or an underlying lymphoma or other malignancy are possible.

The most important investigations would be:

- Blood cultures performed before any antibiotics are given. In this case three blood cultures grew *Streptococcus viridans*.
- Echocardiogram which showed a thickened bicuspid aortic valve, a common congenital abnormality predisposing to significant functional valve disturbance in middle and old age. A transoesophageal echocardiogram is more sensitive in detecting vegetations on the valves.

Treatment with intravenous penicillin and gentamicin for two weeks followed by oral amoxycillin resulted in resolution of the fever with no haemodynamic deterioration or change in the murmurs of mixed aortic valve disease.

After treatment of the endocarditis, the symptoms of pain and tiredness on exertion would need to be considered to see if valve surgery was indicated. Prior to this it would be routine to look at the coronary arteries by angiography to see if simultaneous coronary artery surgery was needed.

✎ KEY POINTS

- Symptoms on exertion in aortic valve disease are a sign that valve surgery needs to be considered.
- In infective endocarditis, it is unusual to have many of the classical physical signs. In the elderly, it may present with non-specific malaise.

A 63-year-old lady is referred to a nephrologist for investigation of polyuria. About four weeks ago she developed abrupt onset extreme thirst and polyuria. She is getting up to pass urine five times a night. Over the past three months she has felt generally unwell and noted pain in her back. She has lost 3 kg in weight over this time. She also has a persistent frontal headache associated with early morning nausea. The headache is worsened by coughing or lying down. Eight years previously she had a left mastectomy and radiotherapy for carcinoma of the breast. She is a retired civil servant who is a non-smoker and drinks 10 units of alcohol per week. She is on no medication.

On examination she is thin and her muscles are wasted. Her pulse rate is 72/min, blood pressure 120/84, jugular venous pressure is not raised, heart sounds are normal and she has no peripheral oedema. Examination of her respiratory, abdominal and neurological systems is normal. Her fundi show papilloedema.

INVESTIGATIONS

		Normal
Haemoglobin	12.2 g/dl	(11.7–15.7 g/dl)
Mean cell volume	85 fl	(80–99 fl)
White cell count	6.7×10^9/l	$(3.5–11.0 \times 10^9$/l)
Platelets	312×10^9/l	$(150–440 \times 10^9$/l)
Sodium	142 mmol/l	(135–145 mmol/l)
Potassium	3.8 mmol/l	(3.5–5.0 mmol/l)
Bicarbonate	26 mmol/l	(24–30 mmol/l)
Urea	4.2 mmol/l	(2.5–6.7 mmol/l)
Creatinine	68 μmol/l	(70–120 μmol/l)
Glucose	4.2 mmol/l	(4.0–6.0 mmol/l)
Albumin	38 g/l	(35–50 g/l)
Calcium	2.75 mmol/l	(2.12–2.65 mmol/l)
Phosphate	1.2 mmol/l	(0.8–1.45 mmol/l)
Bilirubin	12 μmol/l	(3–17 μmol/l)
Alanine transaminase	35 IU/l	(5–35 IU/l)
Alkaline phosphatase	690 IU/l	(30–300 IU/l)
Urinalysis	no protein; no blood	

QUESTIONS

- What is the likely cause of her polyuria?
- How would you investigate and manage this patient?

ANSWER 75

This woman has mild hypercalcaemia but this is not high enough to explain her extreme thirst and polyuria. It is more likely that she has polyuria due to **neurogenic diabetes insipidus as a result of secondary metastases in her hypothalamus**. The hypercalcaemia and raised alkaline phosphatase are suggestive of bony metastases secondary to her breast carcinoma. The recent onset headache, worsened by coughing and lying down and associated with vomiting is characteristic of raised intracranial pressure which is confirmed by the presence of papilloedema. In some tumours around the pituitary there may be compression of the optic nerve causing visual field abnormalities. Neurogenic diabetes insipidus is due to inadequate ADH (antidiuretic hormone arginine vasopressin, AVP) secretion. About 30 per cent of cases of neurogenic diabetes insipidus are idiopathic. The remaining causes are neoplastic, infectious, inflammatory (granulomas), traumatic (neurosurgery; deceleration injury) or vascular (cerebral haemorrhage, infarction). Patients with central diabetes insipidus typically describe an abrupt onset of polyuria and polydipsia. This is because urinary concentration can be maintained fairly well until the number of AVP-secreting neurons in the hypothalamus decreases to 10–15 per cent of the normal number, after which AVP levels decrease to a range where urine output increases dramatically.

! MAJOR CAUSES OF POLYURIA AND POLYDIPSIA

- Solute diuresis, e.g. diabetes mellitus
- Renal diseases which impair urinary concentrating mechanisms e.g. chronic renal failure
- Drinking abnormalities – psychogenic polydipsia
- Renal resistance to the action of AVP:
    nephrogenic diabetes insipidus (due to inherited defects either in the AVP V_2-receptor or the aquaporin-2 receptor)
    hypokalaemia
    hypercalcaemia
    drugs, e.g. lithium, demeclocycline

A water-deprivation test should be performed in this patient measuring the plasma sodium, urine volume and urine osmolality until the sodium rises above 146 mmol/l or the urine osmolality reaches a plateau and the patient has lost at least 2 per cent of body weight. At this point AVP is measured, and the response to subcutaneous desmopressin is measured. An increase in urine osmolality >50 per cent indicates central diabetes insipidus and <10 per cent nephrogenic diabetes insipidus. The hypothalamus should be imaged by MRI scanning and bone X-rays and bone scans performed to identify metastases (Fig. 75.1). The MRI scan (T1-weighted coronal image) through the pituitary shows thickening of the pituitary stalk due to metastatic disease (short arrow) and partial replacement of the normal bone marrow of the clivus by metastatic tumour (long arrow). Treatment of the neurogenic diabetes insipidus involves regular intranasal DDAVP. She should be referred to an oncologist for treatment of her metastatic carcinoma.

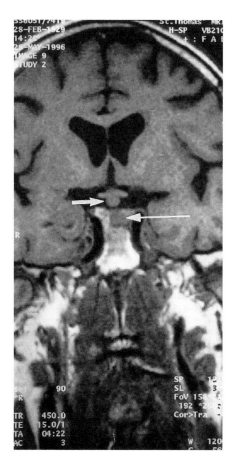

Figure 75.1 MRI scan through pituitary

• The commonest causes of polyuria are diabetes mellitus and chronic renal failure.
• Breast carcinoma may recur after several years of remission.

A 75-year-old man presents with pain in his right thigh and left upper arm. The pain has been present for several months but has become worse. He is otherwise in good health and has had no serious previous medical illnesses. He has become progressively more deaf over the past year but has not sought help for this. The patient is a retired farmer and lives alone. He neither smokes nor drinks alcohol and is taking no regular medication.

On examination, his right leg is bowed laterally. His left humerus appears enlarged and warm. Auditory acuity is markedly reduced in the right ear with reduction in air and bone conduction. Examination is otherwise normal.

INVESTIGATIONS

		Normal
Haemoglobin	13.1 g/dl	(11.7–15.7 g/dl)
Mean cell volume	82 fl	(80–99 fl)
White cell count	8.2 × 10⁹/l	(3.5–11.0 × 10⁹/l)
Platelets	340 × 10⁹/l	(150–440 × 10⁹/l)
Sodium	142 mmol/l	(135–145 mmol/l)
Potassium	4.6 mmol/l	(3.5–5.0 mmol/l)
Urea	4.1 mmol/l	(2.5–6.7 mmol/l)
Creatinine	102 μmol/l	(70–120 μmol/l)
Calcium	2.23 mmol/l	(2.12–2.65 mmol/l)
Phosphate	1.3 mmol/l	(0.8–1.45 mmol/l)
Bilirubin	14 μmol/l	(3–17 μmol/l)
Alanine transaminase	25 IU/l	(5–35 IU/l)
Alkaline phosphatase	584 IU/l	(30–300 IU/l)

QUESTIONS

- What is the likely diagnosis?
- How would you investigate and manage this patient?

ANSWER 76

The combination of a bony abnormality in the leg and arm and nerve deafness with a high alkaline phosphatase suggest that this patient has **Paget's disease** (osteitis deformans). This disease occurs mainly in the elderly and is characterized by excessive and disorganized resorption and formation of bone. Bone pain occurs due to distension of the periosteum, or from deformity causing arthritis. Affected bones are enlarged, deformed and warm. It can affect any bone, but commonly affects the pelvis and spine. The skull is often enlarged and compression of the VIIIth cranial nerve can cause deafness. Rarer complications are high-output cardiac failure secondary to high blood flow through the abnormal bone and osteosarcoma in the affected bone. The major biochemical change is an elevated plasma alkaline phosphatase released by osteoblasts in overactive bone. Serum calcium is usually normal unless the patient is immobilized. The X-ray appearances are of enlarged bone, a resorbing front, thickened and deformed bone and multiple microfractures.

! MAJOR DIFFERENTIAL DIAGNOSES OF BONY PAIN AND DEFORMITY

- Osteomalacia (usually low serum calcium, phosphate, raised alkaline phosphatase)
- Prostatic carcinoma and metastases (raised prostate specific antigen)
- Osteoporosis with fractures (alkaline phosphatase may be raised)
- Fibrous dysplasia

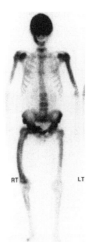

Bone scanning (Fig. 76.1) allows the extent of disease to be assessed and also the effects of treatment to be monitored. Bone scan (using ^{99m}TcMDP) in this patient shows uptake in the right femur, left humerus, pelvis, lumbar spine, skull and scapulae. If osteosarcoma is suspected, a bone biopsy should be performed.

The patient should be given adequate analgesia. Patients only need specific treatment with bisphosphonates or calcitonin if they have severe bone pain, nerve compression or are awaiting orthopaedic surgery. Surgery may be needed for fractures or if there is severe bone pain.

RT   LT

Figure 76.1 Bone scan

⚷ KEY POINTS

- Bony pain and deformity in the elderly may be caused by Paget's disease.
- Rapidly enlarging pagetic bone deformity or severe pain should suggest osteosarcoma.

A 66-year-old man is admitted to hospital with abdominal pain. The abdominal pain started quite suddenly 24 hours before his admission and has continued since then. It is a constant central abdominal pain. He has vomited altered food on one occasion.

He has a history of occasional angina for five years for which he takes a glyceryl trinitrate spray as necessary. This has not been a problem over the last three months. A year ago he was found to be in atrial fibrillation and his GP started him on digoxin, which he still takes. The only other medical history of note is that he has hypertension controlled on a small dose of a thiazide diuretic. He does not take any other medication apart from low-dose aspirin. He used to smoke 10 cigarettes a day but gave up five years ago. He does not drink alcohol. He retired from work as an accountant two years ago.

On examination he was found to be tender with some guarding in the centre of the abdomen. He was in atrial fibrillation at a rate of 88/min with a blood pressure of 116/78. He was admitted to the intensive care unit (ICU) when the blood pressure fell to 84/60 and monitored while initial investigations were performed. The abdominal X-ray showed no gas under the diaphragm and no dilated loops of bowel or fluid levels. While under observation, the urine output falls off. Measurements of cardiac output in ICU showed that it remained high. The observation charts are shown in Fig. 77.1.

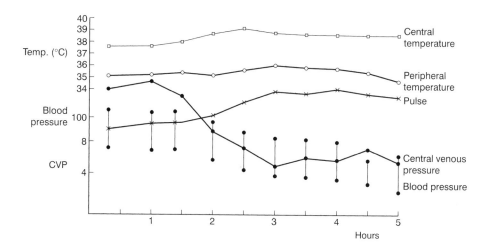

Figure 77.1 ITU chart

- What is the likely cause of the abdominal pain?
- What further developments do the charts suggest?

ANSWER 77

One possibility for the diagnosis of the abdominal pain is **ischaemic bowel** caused by an embolus from the heart. The atrial fibrillation increases the likelihood of such an event. He has been on aspirin which will reduce slightly the risk of embolic events but not on anticoagulants which would have decreased the risk further. In the presence of cardiovascular problems shown by the hypertension and angina anticoagulation would normally be started if there are no contraindications. The risk of cerebrovascular accidents caused by emboli from the heart has been shown to be reduced. In lone atrial fibrillation with no cardiac disease the risks of emboli and the benefits of anticoagulation are less. There are alternative diagnoses such as perforation or pancreatitis and it is not possible to be sure of the cause of the abdominal problem from the information given here.

The chart of the observations covers 10 hours. After the first hour or two the central venous pressure drops, the blood pressure falls and the pulse rate rises in association with the fall in urine output.

These findings show that he is developing shock with inadequate perfusion of vital organs.

! POSSIBLE CAUSES FOR SHOCK

Type of shock	Example
Hypovolaemic shock	Blood loss
Cardiogenic shock	Myocardial infarction
Extracardiac obstructive shock	Pulmonary embolism
Vasodilatory (distributive) shock	Sepsis

All these are possible in this man with abdominal problems and a history of ischaemic heart disease. The fact that the cardiac output is high makes blood loss and cardiogenic shock unlikely. The most likely cause is septic shock where peripheral vasodilatation would lead to a high cardiac output but a falling blood pressure and rising pulse rate. Vasoconstriction and reduced blood flow occurs in certain organs, such as the kidneys, leading to the term 'distributive shock' with maintained overall cardiac output but inappropriate distribution of blood flow. The rise in central temperature and the lack of a marked fall in peripheral temperature would fit with this cause of the shock.

The patient was stabilized with fluid replacement and antibiotics before going to theatre where the diagnosis of ischaemic bowel from an embolus was confirmed.

✎ KEY POINTS

- Aspirin and anticoagulation should be considered in patients with atrial fibrillation.
- Septic shock may be present with warm peripheries through vasodilatation.
- A drop in the central venous pressure may be the first sign of developing shock.

CASE 78

A 52-year-old businessman is referred to a nephrologist for investigation of micro-scopic haematuria. This was first detected six months ago at an insurance medical for a new job, and has since been confirmed on two occasions by his GP. Previous uri-nalyses have been normal. He has never had macroscopic haematuria, and has no uri-nary symptoms. He is otherwise in excellent health. There is no significant past med-ical history. He has no symptoms of visual problems or deafness. There is no family history of renal disease. He drinks 35 units of alcohol per week and smokes 30 ciga-rettes per day.

On examination, he is a fit looking well-nourished man. His pulse is 72/min, blood pressure 146/102. Examination of his cardiovascular, respiratory, abdominal and neu-rological systems is unremarkable. Fundoscopy reveals arteriovenous nipping.

INVESTIGATIONS

		(Normal)
Haemoglobin	13.6 g/dl	(13.3–17.7g/dl)
Mean cell volume	83 fl	(80–99 fl)
White cell count	4.2 × 10⁹/l	(3.9–10.6 × 10⁹/l)
Platelets	213 × 10⁹/l	(150–440 × 10⁹/l)
Sodium	138 mmol/l	(135–145 mmol/l)
Potassium	3.8 mmol/l	(3.5–5.0 mmol/l)
Urea	8.2 mmol/l	(2.5–6.7 mmol/l)
Creatinine	164 μmol/l	(70–120 μmol/l)
Albumin	38 g/l	(35–50g/l)
Glucose	4.5 mmol/l	(4.0–6.0 mmol/l)
Bilirubin	13 μmol/l	(3–17 μmol/l)
Alanine transaminase	33 IU/l	(5–35 IU/l)
Alkaline phosphatase	72 IU/l	(30–300 IU/l)
Gamma-glutamyl transpeptidase	211 IU/l	(11–51 IU/l)

Urinalysis	++ protein; ++ blood; >100 red cells
24-hour urinary protein	1.2 g (< 200 mg/24 h)
ECG	Left ventricular hypertrophy
Renal ultrasound	Two normal sized kidneys

QUESTIONS

- What is the likely diagnosis?
- What further investigations would you organize?
- What advice would you give this patient?

ANSWER 78

Microscopic haematuria has many renal and urological causes (e.g. prostatic disease, stones) but the presence of significant proteinuria, hypertension and renal impairment suggest this man has some form of chronic glomerulonephritis. The high gamma-glutamyl transpeptidase level is compatible with liver disease related to a high alcohol intake. The recommended limit for men is 28 units per week.

! COMMONEST GLOMERULAR CAUSES OF MICROSCOPIC HAEMATURIA

- IgA nephropathy
- Thin basement-membrane disease
- Alport's syndrome

IgA nephropathy is the commonest glomerulonephritis with diffuse mesangial deposits of IgA. Patients often have episodes of macroscopic haematuria concurrent with upper respiratory-tract infection. Most cases of IgA nephropathy are idiopathic, but this type of glomerulonephritis is also commonly associated with Henoch–Schönlein purpura and alcoholic cirrhosis. This man has **IgA nephropathy** in association with alcoholic liver disease. About 20 per cent of patients with IgA nephropathy will develop end-stage renal failure after 20 years of follow-up.

Thin basement-membrane disease is a familial disorder which presents with isolated microscopic haematuria, minimal proteinuria and normal renal function which does not deteriorate. Electron microscopy shows diffuse thinning of the glomerular basement membranes (the width is usually between 150 and 225 nM versus 300–400 nM in normal subjects). Alport's syndrome is a progressive form of glomerular disease, associated with deafness and ocular abnormalities and is usually inherited as an X-linked dominant condition so that males are more seriously affected.

This patient should have a renal biopsy to reach a histological diagnosis. As the patient is over 50 years old he should have urine cytology/prostate-specific antigen/cystoscopy performed to exclude concurrent bladder and prostatic lesions. He needs a liver ultrasound and liver biopsy should be considered.

The patient should be advised to abstain from alcohol, and needs his blood-pressure controlling. He needs regular follow-up as he is at risk of progressing to dialysis and/or renal transplantation. There is no convincing evidence for immunosuppression retarding the progression into renal failure in most patients with IgA nephropathy.

✎ KEY POINTS

- Patients with isolated haematuria aged < 50 years should be initially referred to a nephrologist.
- Patients with isolated haematuria aged > 50 years should be initially referred to a urologist for investigation to exclude bladder or prostatic disease.
- Liver damage from a high alcohol intake may occur with no obvious signs and symptoms.

A 13-year-old Afro-Caribbean patient presents to the casualty department complaining of severe chest pain and shortness of breath. He has had a sore throat for a few days and started developing pain in his back and arms which has increased in severity. Six hours prior to admission he suddenly developed right-sided chest pain which is worse on inspiration and associated with marked breathlessness. He has had previous episodes of pains affecting his fingers and back for which he has taken codeine and ibuprofen. He lives with his parents and is attending school. There is no family history of note.

On examination, he is unwell, febrile 37.8°C and cyanosed. His conjunctivae are pale. Pulse rate is 112/min, regular and blood pressure 136/85. His jugular venous pressure is not raised and heart sounds are normal. His respiratory rate is 28/min and there is a right pleural rub audible. Abdominal and neurological examination is normal.

INVESTIGATIONS

		Normal
Haemoglobin	7.6 g/dl	(13.3–17.7g/dl)
Mean cell volume	86 fl	(80–99 fl)
White cell count	$16.2 \times 10^9/l$	$(3.9–10.6 \times 10^9/l)$
Platelets	$162 \times 10^9/l$	$(150–440 \times 10^9/l)$
Sodium	139 mmol/l	(135–145 mmol/l)
Potassium	4.4 mmol/l	(3.5–5.0 mmol/l)
Urea	6.2 mmol/l	(2.5–6.7 mmol/l)
Creatinine	94 μmol/l	(70–120 μmol/l)
Bicarbonate	24 mmol/l	(24–30 mmol/l)
Arterial blood gases (on air):		
pH	7.33	(7.38–7.44)
pCO_2	2.6 kPa	(4.7–6.0 kPa)
pO_2	7.2 kPa	(12.0–14.5 kPa)
ECG	sinus tachycardia	
Chest X-ray	normal	

QUESTIONS

- What is the likely diagnosis?
- How would you investigate and manage this patient?

ANSWER 79

This boy has **sickle cell disease** and presents with his first serious bony/chest crisis. Sickle cell disease occurs mainly in African negro populations and sporadically in the Mediterranean and Middle East. Haemoglobin S differs from haemoglobin A by the substitution of valine for glutamic acid at position 6 in the β-chain. Sickled cells have increased mechanical fragility and a shortened survival leading to a haemolytic anaemia, and also can block small vessels leading to tissue infarction. Sickle cell disease has a very variable clinical course due to a combination of reasons including the HbF level and socio-economic factors. It usually presents in early childhood with anaemia and jaundice due to a chronic haemolytic anaemia, or painful hands and feet with inflammation of the fingers due to dactylitis. This patient is having a pulmonary crisis characterized by pleuritic chest pain, shortness of breath and hypoxia. It is usually precipitated by dehydration or infection (in this case, a sore throat). The principal differential diagnoses of a patient presenting with pleuritic pain and breathlessness are pneumonia, pneumothorax and pulmonary emboli.

! MAJOR POTENTIAL COMPLICATIONS OF SICKLE CELL DISEASE

- Thrombotic – causing generalized or localized bony pains, abdominal crises, chest crises, neurological signs or priapism
- Aplastic crises – triggered by parvovirus infection
- Haemolytic anaemia
- Sequestration crises in children with rapid enlargement of liver and spleen
- Aseptic necrosis – often of humeral or femoral heads
- Renal failure due to renal medullary infarction or glomerular disease
- Hyposplenism due to autoinfarction in childhood

This patient should be admitted for intravenous fluids, oxygen and adequate analgesia. He has a low arterial pO_2 and appeared cyanosed. Cyanosis is more difficult to see in the presence of anaemia. Infection should be treated with antibiotics. A blood film will show sickled erythrocytes and elevated reticulocyte count. The definitive investigation is haemoglobin electrophoresis which will demonstrate HbS, absent HbA and a variable HbF level. Exchange transfusion may be needed to reduce the level of his sickle cells to less than 30 per cent. He may benefit from long-term hydroxyurea which raises the HbF level and reduces the number of crises.

✎ KEY POINTS

- In Afro-Caribbean patients, sickle cell disease should be thought of as a cause of chest or abdominal pain.
- Patients with sickle cell disease should be looked after in specialized haematology units with psychological support available.

A 66-year-old woman notices that her hands are becoming shaky and is referred to a neurologist. The tremor is worse on the right hand. It is present at rest but is worsened by stress and improved by sleep or using the hand. Alcohol does not seem to help the tremor. Her handwriting has become very small and untidy. She also complains that her muscles feel stiff. She has no significant past medical history. The patient is a retired journalist and lives alone. She does not smoke tobacco and drinks only occasionally. She has hypertension and takes atenolol 50 mg daily.

On examination, the patient has a rather blank facial appearance. Her pulse is 60/min regular, blood pressure 134/84. There are no abnormalities in the cardiovascular or respiratory systems. Her voice is very soft and rather monotonous. There is a tremor affecting mainly her right hand. She has generally increased muscle tone. Power, reflexes, coordination and sensation are normal. Examination of her gait shows that she is slow to get started and has difficulty stopping and turning.

QUESTIONS

- What is the diagnosis?
- How would you investigate and manage this patient?

ANSWER 80

There is evidence in the history and examination of tremor, rigidity and bradykinesia. Her writing shows micrographia secondary to the rigidity and slowness of movement. Her hypertension is well controlled on the beta-blocker. Beta-blockers can cause tiredness and slowness but not to the extent seen in this woman. This woman has **Parkinson's disease** presenting with the classic triad of tremor, rigidity and hypokinesia. Most patients present with tremor which is often unilateral. The combination of tremor and rigidity leads to the cogwheeling rigidity. The patient usually has a blank mask-like facies. There is difficulty starting to walk (freezing) and the patient uses small steps and has difficulty stopping (festination). There is generally normal intellectual function, but there is often depression. The characteristic pathological abnormality is degeneration of dopamine secreting neurons in the nigrostriatal pathway of the basal ganglia.

Parkinsonian features (parkinsonism) may occur in a variety of diseases:

- Parkinson's disease
- Postencephalitic parkinsonism
- Neuroleptic drug-induced parkinson's
- Parkinsonism in association with Alzheimer's/multi-infarct dementia

! CLASSIFICATION OF TREMOR

- Rest tremor. The tremor is worse at rest and is typical of parkinsonism.
- Postural tremor. This is characteristic of benign essential tremor, physiological tremor and exaggerated physiological tremor caused by anxiety, alcohol and thyrotoxicosis. Benign essential tremor is not present at rest, but appears on holding the arms outstretched but is not worse on movement (finger–nose testing). Tests of coordination are normal and walking is unaffected. There is usually a family history of tremor and the tremor is helped by alcohol and beta-blockers.
- Intention tremor. The tremor is worse on movement and is most obvious in finger–nose testing. It is usually caused by brainstem or cerebellar disease caused by such diseases as multiple sclerosis, localized tumours or spinocerebellar degeneration.

The neurologist has a variety of drugs with which to treat this woman's Parkinson's disease. The first-line treatment is selegiline, an inhibitor of monoamine oxidase B which may delay the need to start levodopa and may slow the rate of progression of the disease. Levodopa is usually used in combination with a selective dopa decarboxylase inhibitor which does not cross the blood–brain barrier and reduces peripheral adverse effects. The commonest side-effects are nausea, vomiting, dizziness, postural hypotension and neuropsychiatric problems. After many years of treatment, the patient may develop rapid oscillations in control – the 'on–off' effect. When these develop, a sustained release formulation of levodopa or a dopamine agonist, e.g. bromocriptine may produce improvement. The patient should be assessed by a physiotherapist and occupational therapist and provided with advice and aids. Her house may need to be altered to aid her mobility.

⚷ KEY POINTS

- Parkinson's disease is characterized by tremor, rigidity and hypokinesia.
- Patient management is long term and multidisciplinary.

A 35-year-old accountant is admitted to the casualty department having fainted at home. Over the past six months he has lost 10 kg in weight and has found his appetite is poor. He has been feeling exhausted for several weeks and had difficulty concentrating at work. In the past few days he has had bouts of abdominal pain associated with nausea and vomiting. He has had no previous medical illnesses but had an appendicectomy aged 14. He is married with two children. He is a non-smoker and drinks alcohol very occasionally.

On examination, he looks pale and unwell. There is brown pigmentation of his palmar creases and appendicectomy scar. His pulse rate is 120/min regular, blood pressure 76/36 and jugular venous pressure is not raised. Examination is otherwise normal.

INVESTIGATIONS

		Normal
Haemoglobin	17.2 g/dl	(13.3–17.7g/dl)
Mean cell volume	84 fl	(80–99 fl)
White cell count	7.4 × 10⁹/l	(3.9–10.6 × 10⁹/l)
Platelets	342 × 10⁹/l	(150–440 × 10⁹/l)
Sodium	128 mmol/l	(135–145 mmol/l)
Potassium	5.7 mmol/l	(3.5–5.0 mmol/l)
Urea	15.2 mmol/l	(2.5–6.7 mmol/l)
Creatinine	116 μmol/l	(70–120 μmol/l)
Albumin	48 g/l	(35–50g/l)
Glucose	2.3 mmol/l	(4.0–6.0 mmol/l)
Urinalysis	no protein; no blood; no glucose	
ECG	sinus tachycardia	
Chest X-ray	normal	

QUESTIONS

- What is the diagnosis?
- How would you investigate and manage this patient?

ANSWER 81

This patient has marked weight loss.

❗ CAUSES OF WEIGHT LOSS

- With an increased appetite
  diabetes mellitus
  thyrotoxicosis
  malabsorption
- With a poor appetite
  malignancy
  chronic infection, e.g. tuberculosis
  endocrine causes, e.g. Addison's disease, panhypopituitarism
  cardiac, respiratory, renal failure
  psychiatric causes, e.g. anorexia nervosa

This patient has features characteristic of **acute adrenal insufficiency (Addison's disease)** with shock. The typical symptoms of adrenal failure are nausea, anorexia, weight loss, tiredness, weakness and pigmentation of skin creases. An addisonian crisis may be precipitated by some minor illness or surgery. Mineralocorticoid (aldosterone) deficiency causes sodium and water depletion. During a crisis, excess antidiuretic hormone (ADH) is secreted leading to hyponatraemia. Hyperkalaemia and metabolic acidosis occur due to lack of potassium secretion in the distal tubule. The fluid depletion leads to a reduced glomerular filtration rate and a moderately raised blood urea concentration. Glucocorticoid deficiency leads to hypoglycaemia. Primary hypoadrenalism is due to adrenal destruction either by autoimmune adrenalitis, tuberculosis, metastatic carcinoma, infarction or amyloidosis. Secondary hypoadrenalism is commonly due to adrenal suppression by exogenous steroids or more rarely by hypothalamic/pituitary pathology.

This patient should have blood taken for a random blood cortisol level. In any acutely ill patient without adrenal failure the plasma cortisol is normally > 600 nmol/l. In primary adrenal failure, there will be an elevated adrenocorticotrophic hormone (ACTH) level as well as a low cortisol. If there is any doubt about the diagnosis an ACTH-stimulation test should be done at a later stage. Normally the plasma cortisol rises to 600–1300 nmol/l at 1h, and 1000–1800 nmol/l at 2h. Adrenal autoantibodies should be measured. In this case there is a need for urgent treatment with intravenous hydrocortisone, intravenous glucose and rapid fluid replacement with intravenous saline. This should be started on the basis of the clinical picture given here without waiting for confirmation from cortisol levels. He will require long term adrenal hormone replacement with prednisolone and fludrocortisone. He should carry a steroid-dependency card and increase his dose of prednisolone in the event of a fever or intercurrent illness.

✎ KEY POINTS

- Adrenal insufficiency causes profound sodium and water depletion.
- An addisonian crisis may be precipitated by infection, myocardial infarction, surgery or any metabolic stress.

A 50-year-old woman complains to her GP of rectal bleeding. She has noticed this problem over the last three months. She has always had a tendency to be constipated and this has become more of a problem recently. She takes bran intermittently to try to control it. She says that she often has to strain to pass her bowel motions and this has been causing her some pain over the last three weeks. She has noticed that blood occasionally drips into the toilet bowl. When she wipes herself she has found streaks of blood on the toilet paper on several occasions.

She has no other symptoms and has not been to the surgery for over ten years. Her appetite is good and she has put on 5 kg in weight over the last year. She is a non-smoker and non-drinker. There is a family history of thyroid disease in her mother and her sister. She works as a secretary. She is married with two grown-up children.

On examination, there is nothing abnormal to find on examination of the abdomen or any other system.

INVESTIGATIONS

		Normal
Haemoglobin	12.6 g/dl	11.7–15.7 g/dl
Mean corpuscular volume (MCV)	89 fl	80.8–100.0 fl
White cell count	$6.5 \times 10^9/l$	$3.5–11.0 \times 10^9/l$
Platelet count	$280 \times 10^9/l$	$150–440 \times 10^9/l$

QUESTIONS

- Are any further investigations indicated?
- What is the most likely diagnosis?

ANSWER 82

The story is one of constipation, straining to pass motions and blood in the pan and on the toilet paper. The most likely diagnosis is that she has **haemorrhoids**. However, the recent onset of rectal bleeding in a patient over the age of 40 should always be taken seriously even if the bleeding is typical of haemorrhoids.

There is a move towards screening for occult large bowel carcinoma which responds well to removal if detected early enough.

The story of constipation, the weight increase over the last year and the family history of thyroid disease raise the possibility that she might have hypothyroidism as an underlying cause of the constipation. There is no other clue in the blood count where hypothyroidism can produce a high mean corpuscular volume or even a macrocytic anaemia. The thyroid function tests should be checked. This could be done by a measurement of thyroid-stimulating hormone which would be raised in hypothyroidism.

Further investigation to rule out any other lesion in the left side of the colon is necessary. Rectal examination is not mentioned in the text and a careful examination including proctoscopy to look for haemorrhoids should be performed. In addition she should have a sigmoidoscopy to make sure that there is no other lesion in the sigmoid colon and no sign of any blood coming from higher up. It is dangerous to assume that the bleeding is all related to haemorrhoids even if these are found at proctoscopy.

KEY POINTS

- Rectal bleeding needs investigation even if there is evidence of a possible peri-anal cause.
- Bleeding from haemorrhoids provides a typical story of streaking on the outside of the motion or on the toilet paper.

A 16-year-old boy is referred to hospital because jaundice has been noticed. He has developed malaise and anorexia over six months and the jaundice has been evident for the last week. He is a non-smoker and he denies any alcohol consumption. He has not been on any prescribed treatment and denies any other drug ingestion or administration.

Apart from common childhood illnesses he has no relevant medical history. He has had a normal vaccination programme. There is a suggestion from his father that an uncle may have died in his teens from liver disease but there is no other relevant family history.

When he entered secondary school he was performing adequately in the lower half of his class. His results have steadily deteriorated and his parents have been worried by difficulties at home and at school with his work and his behaviour.

On examination he is jaundiced. There are no abnormal signs in the abdomen, cardiovascular or respiratory systems. In the nervous system he is found to have some abnormal movements on examination of the limbs but power and reflexes are normal. He seems slow and formal psychological testing is arranged. This shows that he has an IQ of 80.

INVESTIGATIONS

		Normal
Sodium	140 mmol/l	(135–145 mmol/l)
Potassium	4.5 mmol/l	(3.5–5.0 mmol/l)
Urea	3.6 mmol/l	(2.5–6.7 mmol/l)
Creatinine	69 μmol/l	(70–120 μmol/l)
Calcium	2.28 mmol/l	(2.12–2.65 mmol/l)
Phosphate	1.16 mmol/l	(0.8–1.45 mmol/l)
Total bilirubin	46 μmol/l	(3–17 μmol/l)
Alkaline phosphatase	534 IU/l	(30–300 IU/l)
Alanine aminotransferase	136 IU/l	(5–35 IU/l)
Gamma-glutamyl transpeptidase	78 IU/l	(11–51IU)

QUESTION

- What is the likely diagnosis and how might it be confirmed?

ANSWER 83

The picture of hepatic abnormality, neurological signs and intellectual deterioration is likely to represent **Wilson's disease (hepatolenticular degeneration)**. This is an autosomal recessive disease in which copper accumulates in the liver and the brain. There is progressive development of extrapyramidal signs and dementia. The hepatic picture is variable but may progress to cirrhosis of the liver. Such a diagnosis should always be considered in a young person who develops liver disease. The liver disease is usually evident by this age.

The neurological problems are most often extrapyramidal features such as the abnormal movements in this boy and slowly progressive dementia. Diagnosis at an early stage is important because of the possibility of treatment to halt the deterioration.

The diagnosis can be made on the finding of copper accumulation in a liver biopsy, decreased caeruloplasmin in the serum, increased urinary copper excretion and the presence of Kayser–Fleischer rings which are visible on slit-lamp examination of the cornea. These are brown or grey deposits of copper in Descemet's membrane. They are most marked in the upper part of the circumference and can be seen by an experienced observer with a hand lens and adequate lighting.

Treatment is with oral penicillamine which chelates copper and increases its urinary excretion. If this diagnosis is confirmed then any young relatives should be screened by regular liver-function tests and neurological examination so that treatment can be started before significant hepatic, neurological and psychological changes develop. Prognosis is improved considerably by early diagnosis and treatment.

✎ KEY POINTS

- There are certain uncommon disorders which are important despite their rarity because they present in a variety of ways and early diagnosis is crucial in the prevention of irreversible damage.
- Diagnostic signs such as Kayser–Fleischer rings are only observed if specifically sought once the diagnosis has been suspected.

CASE 84

A 67-year-old woman, a lifelong non-smoker, presents with shortness of breath and ankle oedema. She has a story of gradually increasing shortness of breath over two years but has never sought help for any respiratory problems. Over the past four years she has noticed increasing pain in the knees. She was seen in a rheumatology clinic and was told that she had degenerative changes caused by osteoarthritis. She had a cholecystectomy 15 years previously. She is on no treatment except that she takes occasional paracetamol and ibuprofen which she buys from her local chemist.

On examination the pulse is 80/min, blood pressure is 132/86. The respiratory rate is 18/min. The jugular venous pressure is raised 5 cm and there is oedema up to the mid-calf level. On auscultation of the chest she has expiratory polyphonic wheezes but no crackles.

Chest X-ray and respiratory function-tests are performed

RESPIRATORY FUNCTION TEST

	Actual	Post-salbutamol	Predicted
FEV_1 (l)	0.50	0.85	2.4–3.0
FVC (l)	2.02	2.40	3.2–4.0
FER (FEV_1/FVC) (%)	25	35	72–78
PEF (l/min)	80	135	360–440
T_LCO (mmol/kPa/min)	6.0		9.2
V_A (l)	3.0		4.8
K_{CO} (mmol/kPa/min/l)	2.0		1.8
PaO_2 (kPa)	5.0		10–13.3
$PaCO_2$ (kPa)	5.2		4.8–6.1

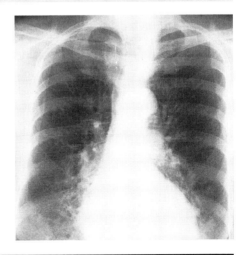

Figure 84.1 Chest X-ray

QUESTIONS

- What is the most likely explanation of these findings?
- What should be the management of this woman?

ANSWER 84

This 67-year-old woman has severe airflow obstruction with a small but significant immediate response to a bronchodilator. She has evidence of right heart failure and the blood gases show severe hypoxia sufficient to produce this problem.

In the absence of a smoking history, chronic obstructive pulmonary disease (COPD) is unlikely. It might occur in association with a hereditary problem such as α_1-antitrypsin deficiency producing emphysema. Although the chest X-ray shows overinflation (right hemidiaphragm is down to below the seventh rib anteriorly in the midclavicular line) the normal to high K_{co} (diffusion coefficient, transfer factor per unit of lung volume calculated from T_Lco/V_A) is against the diagnosis of emphysema where breakdown of the alveolar capillary membrane causes a low transfer factor (T_Lco) and K_{co}. Rheumatoid arthritis can produce a rare form of alveolar obstruction called obliterative bronchiolitis but her joint problem appears to be osteoarthritis. The most likely explanation is that she has **chronic asthma** which has never been diagnosed and treated. Around 15–20 per cent of asthmatics have a very poor perception of their airway narrowing. The use of a non-steroidal anti-inflammatory drug might contribute since around 5 per cent of asthmatics are sensitive to aspirin and non-steroidals which increase airway obstruction, probably through their inhibition of prostaglandin synthetase increasing leukotriene formation.

This woman was given diuretics and continuous low-flow oxygen initially together with inhaled bronchodilators and prednisolone at a dose of 30 mg daily. Her ibuprofen was stopped. Her airflow obstruction improved over two weeks to an FEV_1 of 1.8 l and an FVC of 2.8 l. Oxygen and diuretics were stopped and her improvement was maintained with inhaled steroids regularly and inhaled β_2-agonists as needed. The failure to return to normal levels of lung function suggests irreversible damage from the chronic uncontrolled asthma.

✎ KEY POINTS

- A vigorous attempt should always be made to reverse moderate-to-severe obstruction.
- In COPD around 10 per cent of cases have a significant steroid response compared to the great majority of asthmatics.
- Aspirin and non-steroidal anti-inflammatory drugs can provoke asthma.
- Diffusion coefficient (T_Lco/V_A) is low in emphysema but normal or slightly high in asthma.

CASE 85

The medical team are asked to review a postoperative surgical patient. A 62-year-old lady had been admitted 10 days previously to have a right hemicolectomy performed for a caecal carcinoma. This was discovered on colonoscopy which was performed to investigate an iron-deficiency anaemia and change in bowel habit. She is otherwise fit with no significant medical history. She is a retired teacher. She neither smokes, nor drinks alcohol and is on no medication. Her pre-operative serum creatinine was 76 μmol/l. The initial surgery was uneventful, and she was given cefuroxime and metronidazole as routine antibiotic prophylaxis. However the patient developed a prolonged ileus associated with abdominal pain. On postoperative day 5, the patient started to spike fevers up to 38.5°C and was commenced on intravenous gentamicin 80 mg t.d.s. in addition to the other antibiotics. Over the next five days the patient remained persistently febrile, with negative blood cultures. In the last 24 hours, she had also become relatively hypotensive with her systolic blood pressure being about 95 mmHg despite intravenous colloids. Her urine output is now 15 ml/h.

On examination the lady is unwell and sweating profusely. She is jaundiced. Her pulse rate is 110/min regular, blood pressure 95/60 and jugular venous pressure is not raised. Her heart sounds are normal. Her respiratory rate is 30/min. Her breath sounds are normal. Her abdomen is tender with guarding over the right iliac fossa. Bowel sounds are absent.

INVESTIGATIONS

		Normal
Haemoglobin	8.2 g/dl	(11.7–15.7 g/dl)
Mean cell volume	83 fl	(80–99 fl)
White cell count	26.3 × 10⁹/l	(3.5–11.0 × 10⁹/l)
Platelets	94 × 10⁹/l	(150–440 × 10⁹/l)
Sodium	126 mmol/l	(135–145 mmol/l)
Potassium	5.8 mmol/l	(3.5–5.0 mmol/l)
Bicarbonate	6 mmol/l	(24–30 mmol/l)
Urea	36.2 mmol/l	(2.5–6.7 mmol/l)
Creatinine	523 μmol/l	(70–120 μmol/l)
Glucose	2.6 mmol/l	(4.0–6.0 mmol/l)
Albumin	31 g/l	(35–50g/l)
Bilirubin	95 μmol/l	(3–17 μmol/l)
Alanine transaminase	63 IU/l	(5–35 IU/l)
Alkaline phosphatase	363 IU/l	(30–300 IU/l)
Trough gentamicin level	4.8 μg/ml	(<2.0 μg/ml)
Urinalysis	+blood;+protein; granular casts and epithelial cells	

QUESTIONS

- What are the causes of this patient's renal failure?
- How would you further investigate and manage this patient?

ANSWER 85

This patient has postoperative acute renal failure due to a combination of **intra-abdominal sepsis and aminoglycoside nephrotoxicity**. Her sepsis is due to an anastomotic leak with a localized peritonitis which has been partially controlled with antibiotics. Her sepsis syndrome is manifested by fever, tachycardia, hypotension, hypoglycaemia, metabolic acidosis (low bicarbonate) and oliguria. The low sodium and high potassium are common in this condition as cell membrane function becomes less effective. The elevated white count is a marker for bacterial infection and the low platelet count is part of the picture of disseminated intravascular coagulation. Jaundice and abnormal liver-function tests are common features of intra-abdominal sepsis. Aminoglycosides (gentamicin, streptomycin, amikacin) cause auditory and vestibular dysfunction, as well as acute renal failure. Risk factors for aminoglycoside nephrotoxicity are higher doses and duration of treatment, increased age, pre-existing renal insufficiency, hepatic failure and volume depletion. Aminoglycoside nephrotoxicity usually occurs 7–10 days after starting treatment. Monitoring of trough levels is important although an increase in the trough level generally indicates decreased excretion of the drug caused by a fall in the glomerular flow rate. Thus, nephrotoxicity is already established by the time the trough level rises.

This patient needs urgent resuscitation. She requires transfer to the intensive care unit where she will need invasive circulatory monitoring with a pulmonary artery catheter to allow accurate assessment of her colloid and inotrope requrements. She also needs urgent renal replacement therapy to correct her acidosis and hyperkalaemia. In a haemodynamically unstable patient like this, continuous haemofiltration is the preferred method. The patient also needs urgent surgical review. The abdomen should be imaged with either ultrasound or computed tomography (CT) scanning to try to identify any collection of pus. Once haemodynamically stable, the patient should have a laparotomy to drain any collection and form a temporary colostomy.

KEY POINTS

- Postoperative acute renal failure is often multifactorial due to hypotension, sepsis and nephrotoxic drugs such as aminoglycosides and NSAIDs.
- Sepsis syndrome must be recognized early and treated aggressively to reduce the morbidity and mortality of this condition.

A 62-year-old man is receiving chemotherapy for non-Hogkin's lymphoma which was diagnosed four months previously. Three weeks prior to this admission he spiked a fever up to 38.5°C, and blood cultures grew *Staphylococcus aureus*. His Hickman line (through which chemotherapy was given) was removed and he was treated with a single dose of intravenous vancomycin. He has now been admitted with severe neck pain which is worse on turning his head. He feels unwell and has been shivering and having rigors. Over the past 24 hours he has noted difficulty walking and now he has lost all power and sensation in his arms and legs. He is a retired bus driver. He smokes 15 cigarettes a day and drinks 10 units of alcohol per week. He is on two antihypertensive agents.

On examination, he is febrile 38.5°C. His pulse is 116/min regular and blood pressure 92/66. His heart sounds are normal. His respiratory and abdominal systems are normal. He is acutely tender over his cervical spine. The patient is able to slightly abduct his shoulders but otherwise has no power in his arms and legs. His tendon reflexes are absent. Sensation is absent below the sternal notch. He is tender over his lower cervical spine. The cranial nerves are normal.

INVESTIGATIONS

		Normal
Haemoglobin	14.6 g/dl	(13.3–17.7g/dl)
Mean cell volume	85 fl	(80–99fl)
White cell count	18.6×10^9/l	($3.9–10.6 \times 10^9$/l)
Platelets	412×10^9/l	($150–440 \times 10^9$/l)
Erythrocyte sedimentation rate	74 mm/h	(<10 mm/h)
Sodium	138 mmol/l	(135–145 mmol/l)
Potassium	4.6 mmol/l	(3.5–5.0 mmol/l)
Urea	4.2 mmol/l	(2.5–6.7 mmol/l)
Creatinine	74 μmol/l	(70–120 μmol/l)
Bilirubin	14 μmol/l	(3–17 μmol/l)
Alanine transaminase	16 IU/l	(5–35 IU/l)
Alkaline phosphatase	453 IU/l	(30–300 IU/l)

QUESTIONS

- What is the likely diagnosis and major differential diagnoses?
- How would you investigate and manage this patient?

ANSWER 86

The most likely diagnosis is that this man has **staphylococcal osteomyelitis** affecting his cervical spine with an epidural abscess causing acute spinal cord compression and tetraplegia. The staphylococcal infection has seeded to his cervical spine following his bacteraemia three weeks previously and inadequate antibiotic treatment. The clinical picture is that of rapidly advancing paraplegia and local tenderness at the site of the abscess. The patient has signs of bacterial infection with fever, tachycardia, hypotension and neutrophil leukocytosis. The raised alkaline phosphatase suggests bony destruction. Patients at high risk of osteomyelitis are those with trauma, rheumatoid arthritis, indwelling vascular catheters, intravenous drug addicts and patients receiving chemotherapy and immunosuppression.

! DIFFERENTIAL DIAGNOSIS OF CORD COMPRESSION

- Trauma
- Benign tumour e.g. meningioma, neurofibroma
- Rheumatoid arthritis – spontaneous dislocation of cervical vertebrae
- Spontaneous epidural haemorrhage (anticoagulants)
- Metastatic vertebral deposits
- Spinal tuberculosis

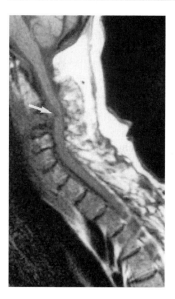

This patient had urgent imaging of his cervical spine with MRI scanning (Fig. 86.1). MRI cervical spine demonstrated spinal cord compression (arrow) at the level of C3/C4. The epidural abscess was drained surgically and appropriate antibiotics were continued for six weeks. A bone scan is helpful in this situation to detect other sites of osteomyelitis.

Figure 86.1 MRI scan of cervical spine

⚲ KEY POINTS

- Staphylococcal osteomyelitis is a common cause of back pain in certain high risk patients.
- It can progress to spinal cord compression and spinal artery thrombosis and is therefore a medical emergency.

A 67-year-old man attends his GP's surgery. He says that he has lost 10 kg in weight over the last four months. This has been associated with a decrease in appetite and an increasing problem with vomiting. The vomiting has been productive of food eaten many hours previously.

He is a smoker of 20 cigarettes per day and drinks around 10 units of alcohol each week. There is no relevant family history. His past medical history consists of hypertension which was treated for two years with beta-blockers. He stopped taking these four months ago.

On examination, he looks thin and unwell. His pulse is 82/min. There are no abnormalities to find on examination of the cardiovascular and respiratory systems. There are no masses to feel in the abdomen and no tenderness but a succussion splash is present. His blood pressure is 148/86. The chest X-ray is clear.

INVESTIGATIONS

		Normal
Sodium	130 mmol/l	(135–145 mmol/l)
Potassium	3.0 mmol/l	(3.5–5.0 mmol/l)
Chloride	82 mmol/l	(95–105 mmol/l)
Bicarbonate	41 mmol/l	(25–35 mmol/l)
Urea	15.6 mmol/l	(2.5–6.7 mmol/l)
Creatinine	100 μmol/l	(76–120 μmol/l)
Calcium	2.38 mmol/l	(2.12–2.65 mmol/l)
Phosphate	1.16 mmol/l	(0.8–1.45 mmol/l)
Alkaline phosphatase	128 IU/l	(30–300 IU/l)
Alanine aminotransferase	32 IU/l	(5–35 IU/l)
Gamma-glutamyl transpeptidase	38 IU/l	(11–51 IU/l)

QUESTIONS

- What is the likely explanation for these findings?
- What is the most likely diagnosis?

ANSWER 87

The clinical picture suggests **obstruction to outflow from the stomach**. This would be compatible with vomiting of residual food some time after eating and the succussion splash from the retained fluid and food in the stomach. The biochemical results fit with this diagnosis. There is a greater rise in urea than creatinine suggesting a degree of dehydration. Sodium, chloride and hydrogen ions are lost in the vomited stomach contents. Loss of hydrochloric acid produces a metabolic alkalosis. In compensation, hydrogen ions are exchanged for potassium in the kidney and across the cell membranes, and carbonic acid dissociates to hydrogen ions and bicarbonate.

The most likely cause would be a carcinoma of the stomach involving the pyloric antrum to give obstruction to outflow. A chronic gastric ulcer in this area could produce the same picture from associated scarring and gastroscopy and biopsy would be necessary to be sure of the diagnosis.

Gastroscopy may be difficult because of retained food in the stomach. In this case, after this was washed out a tumour was visible at the pylorus causing almost complete obstruction of the outflow tract of the stomach. The next step would be a computed tomography (CT) scan of the abdomen to look for filling defects in the liver and any suggestion of local spread of the tumour outside the stomach. If there is no evidence of extension or spread, or even to relieve obstruction, laparotomy and resection should be considered. Otherwise chemotherapy and surgical palliation are options in treatment.

✎ KEY POINTS

- Vomiting food eaten a long time previously suggests gastric outlet obstruction.
- Mild-to-moderate dehydration tends to increase urea more than creatinine.
- Prolonged vomiting causes a typical picture of hypochloraemic metabolic alkalosis.

CASE 88

A 63-year-old woman goes to her GP complaining of extreme tiredness. She has been increasingly fatigued over the past year but in recent weeks she has become breathless on exertion, light-headed and complained of headaches. Her feet have become numb and she has started to become unsteady on her feet. She has had no significant previous medical illnesses. She is a retired teacher and lives alone. She is a non-smoker and drinks about 15 units of alcohol per week. She is taking no regular medication. Her mother and one of her two sisters have thyroid problems.

On examination, her conjunctivae are pale and sclerae are yellow. Her temperature is 37.8°C. Her pulse rate is 96/min regular and blood pressure 142/72. Examination of her heart, respiratory and abdominal systems is normal. She has a symmetrical distal weakness affecting her arms and legs. Knee and ankle jerks are absent and she has extensor plantar responses. She has sensory loss in a glove and stocking distribution with a particularly severe loss of joint position sense.

BLOOD TESTS

		Normal
Haemoglobin	4.2 g/dl	(11.7–15.7 g/dl)
Mean cell volume	112 fl	(80–99 fl)
White cell count	3.3 × 10⁹/l	(3.5–11.0 × 10⁹/l)
Platelets	102 × 10⁹/l	(150–440 × 10⁹/l)
Sodium	136 mmol/l	(135–145 mmol/l)
Potassium	4.4 mmol/l	(3.5–5.0 mmol/l)
Urea	5.2 mmol/l	(2.5–6.7 mmol/l)
Creatinine	92 µmol/l	(70–120 µmol/l)
Glucose	4.4 mmol/l	(4.0–6.0 mmol/l)
Bilirubin	45 µmol/l	(3–17 µmol/l)
Alanine transaminase	33 IU/l	(5–35 IU/l)
Alkaline phosphatase	263 IU/l	(30–300 IU/l)

QUESTIONS

- What is the diagnosis?
- How would you investigate and manage this patient?

ANSWER 88

This patient has a severe macrocytic anaemia and neurological signs due to **vitamin B$_{12}$ deficiency**. There is a family history of thyroid disease. This can cause a macrocytic anaemia but not to this degree and hypothyroidism would not explain the other features. Anaemia reduces tissue oxygenation and therefore can affect most organ systems. The symptoms and signs of anaemia depend on its rapidity of onset. Chronic anaemia causes fatigue and pallor of the mucous membranes. Cardiorespiratory symptoms and signs include breathlessness, chest pain, claudication, tachycardia, oedema and other signs of cardiac failure. Gastrointestinal symptoms include anorexia, weight loss, nausea and constipation. There may be menstrual irregularities and loss of libido. Neurological symptoms include headache, dizziness and cramps. There may be a low-grade fever. In pernicious anaemia, the mean cell volume can rise to 100–140 fl and oval macrocytes are seen on the blood film. The reticulocyte count is inappropriately low for the degree of anaemia. The white cell count is usually moderately reduced. There is often a mild rise in serum bilirubin giving the patient a 'lemon-yellow' complexion. As in this patient, profound vitamin B$_{12}$ deficiency also causes a peripheral neuropathy and subacute degeneration of the posterior columns and pyramidal tracts in the spinal cord causing a sensory loss and increased difficulty walking. The peripheral neuropathy and pyramidal tract involvement produce the combination of absent ankle jerks and upgoing plantars. In its most extreme form it can lead to paraplegia, optic atrophy and dementia. Vitamin B$_{12}$ is synthesized by microorganisms and is obtained by ingesting animal or vegetable products contaminated by bacteria. After ingestion, it is bound by intrinsic factor synthesized by gastric parietal cells and this complex is then absorbed in the terminal ileum. Vitamin B$_{12}$ deficiency is most commonly due to a gastric cause (pernicious anaemia due to an autoimmune atrophic gastritis; total gastrectomy), bacterial overgrowth in the small intestine destroying intrinsic factor or a malabsorption from the terminal ileum (surgical resection; Crohn's disease).

! DIFFERENTIAL DIAGNOSES OF MACROCYTIC ANAEMIA

- Folate deficiency
- Excessive alcohol consumption
- Hypothyroidism
- Certain drugs, e.g. azathioprine, methotrexate
- Primary acquired sideroblastic anaemia and myelodysplastic syndromes

A full dietary history should be taken. Vegans who omit all animal products from their diet often have subclinical vitamin B$_{12}$ deficiency. Serum vitamin B$_{12}$ and folate levels should be measured and antibodies to intrinsic factor and parietal cells should be assayed. Intrinsic factor antibodies are virtually specific for pernicious anaemia but are only present in about 50 per cent of cases. Parietal cell antibody is present in 85–90 per cent of patients with pernicious anaemia but can also occur in patients with other causes of atrophic gastritis. A radioactive B$_{12}$ absorption test (Schilling test) distinguishes gastric from intestinal causes of deficiency. Rapid correction of vitamin B$_{12}$

is essential using intramuscular hydroxycobalamin to prevent cardiac failure and further neurological damage.

CASE 89

A 45-year-old publican suffered a subendocardial inferior myocardial infarction four months previously which was treated with thrombolytics and aspirin. He continued to develop angina and coronary angiography was performed. This showed severe triple-vessel disease and he had coronary artery bypass grafting performed. He now attends a cardiac rehabilitation clinic. He has had no further angina since his surgery. He has a strong family history of ischaemic heart disease with his father and two paternal uncles having died of myocardial infarctions in their fifties. He is married with two children. He smokes 25 cigarettes per day and drinks 40 units of alcohol per week. His medication is atenolol and aspirin.

On examination, he is slightly overweight (85 kg; body mass index=28). He has nicotine-stained nails. He has bilateral corneal arcus, xanthelasmata around his eyes and xanthomata on his Achilles tendons. He has a well-healed midline sternotomy scar. His pulse is 64/min regular, blood pressure 150/84. He has no palpable pedal pulses. His respiratory, gastrointestinal and neurological systems are normal.

INVESTIGATIONS

		Normal
Haemoglobin	16.2 g/dl	(13.3–17.7g/dl)
White cell count	10.2. × 10⁹/l	(3.9–10.6 × 10⁹/l)
Platelets	237 × 10⁹/l	(150–440 × 10⁹/l)
Sodium	136 mmol/l	(135–145 mmol/l)
Potassium	3.8 mmol/l	(3.5–5.0 mmol/l)
Urea	3.6 mmol/l	(2.5–6.7 mmol/l)
Creatinine	82 μmol/l	(70–120 μmol/l)
Bilirubin	13 μmol/l	(3–17 μmol/l)
Alanine transaminase	33 IU/l	(5–35 IU/l)
Alkaline phosphatase	72 IU/l	(30–300 IU/l)
Cholesterol	12.2 mmol/l	(3.9–7.8 mmol/l)
Triglyceride	2.30 mmol/l	(0.55–1.90 mmol/l)
VLDL*	0.34 mmol/l	(0.12–0.65 mmol/l)
LDL*	8.5 mmol/l	(1.6–4.4 mmol/l)
HDL*	0.6 mmol/l	(0.9–1.9 mmol/l)
Urinalysis	NAD	

*Abbreviations: VLDL = very low density lipoprotein; LDL = low density lipoprotein; HDL = high density lipoprotein

QUESTIONS

- What is the metabolic abnormality present?
- What advice would you give this man?

The obvious abnormal investigation is a very high serum cholesterol with high LDL and low HDL levels. He has many clinical features to go with the high cholesterol and premature vascular disease. This man has **familial hypercholesterolaemia**. He has presented with premature coronary artery disease. His absent pedal pulses suggest peripheral vascular disease. Familial hypercholesterolaemia is an autosomal dominant condition. The homozygous condition is rare and affected individuals usually die before the age of 20 years due to premature atherosclerosis. The heterozygous form affects about 1 in 400 individuals in the UK, and 50 per cent of males will develop ischaemic heart disease before the age of 50 years. Corneal arcus, xanthelasmata and xanthomata on Achilles tendons and the extensor tendons on the dorsum of the hands develop in early adult life. The metabolic defect is a result of a reduced number of high-affinity cell-surface LDL receptors. This leads to increased LDL levels. Increased uptake of LDL by macrophage scavenger receptors leads to increased oxidized LDL which is particularly atherogenic. Triglyceride and VLDL levels are normal or mildly elevated. HDL levels are low. The other major causes of hypercholesterolaemia are familial combined hyperlipidaemia and polygenic hypercholesterolaemia. Familial combined hyperlipidaemia differs from familial hypercholesterolaemia by patients having raised triglycerides. Patients with polygenic hypercholesterolaemia have a similar lipid profile to familial hypercholesterolaemia but they do not develop xanthomata. Hypercholesterolaemia may commonly occur in the following medical conditions – hypothyroidism, diabetes mellitus, nephrotic syndrome and hepatic cholestasis.

This patient is at extremely high risk for further vascular events and especially occlusion of his coronary artery bypass grafts. He should be advised to stop smoking, reduce his alcohol intake, take more exercise and eat a strict low cholesterol diet. Diet alone will not control his cholesterol. He should have pharmacological treatment with a HMG CoA reductase inhibitor and a bile acid sequestrant. His children should have their lipid profile measured so that they can be treated to prevent premature coronary artery disease. There is clear evidence from clinical trials that primary prevention of coronary artery disease can be achieved by lowering serum cholesterol. The West of Scotland Coronary Prevention Study (WOSCOPS) showed cholesterol lowering with pravastatin reduced both the number of coronary events and coronary mortality in middle age men with a serum LDL level of greater than 4 mmol/l.

✎ KEY POINTS

- The commonest causes for hypercholesterolaemia are polygenic hypercholesterolaemia, familial hypercholesterolaemia and familial combined hyperlipidaemia.
- Effective drugs are now available to treat hypercholesterolaemia and should be used aggressively to reduce coronary artery disease.

CASE 90

A 46-year-old man is referred to a gastroenterologist by his GP complaining of severe persistent epigastric pain. The pain is worse before a meal and is partially relieved by antacids. Three months previously the GP organized an upper gastrointestinal endoscopy which showed a posterior duodenal ulcer. Biopsies showed no evidence of *Helicobacter pylori* infection. The patient was started on ranitidine 150 mg b.d. which he remains on. The patient feels increasingly fatigued, and his motions have become increasingly loose. He has had no other serious medical illnesses. He is a taxi driver and married with three children. He smokes 20 cigarettes a day and drinks about 25 units of alcohol per week.

On examination, the patient looks well but his conjunctivae are pale. His pulse is 72/min and blood pressure 118/78. He is tender in the epigastrium. There are no masses palpable. Physical examination is otherwise normal. The gastroenterologist organizes the following blood tests.

BLOOD TESTS

		Normal
Haemoglobin	8.7 g/dl	(13.3–17.7g/dl)
Mean cell volume	71 fl	(80–99 fl)
White cell count	5.6 × 10⁹/l	(3.9–10.6 × 10⁹/l)
Platelets	342 × 10⁹/l	(150–440 × 10⁹/l)
Sodium	137 mmol/l	(135–145 mmol/l)
Potassium	4.8 mmol/l	(3.5–5.0 mmol/l)
Urea	5.2 mmol/l	(2.5–6.7 mmol/l)
Creatinine	124 μmol/l	(70–150 μmol/l)
Albumin	39 g/l	(35–50g/l)
Glucose	4.7 mmol/l	(4.0–6.0 mmol/l)
Bilirubin	12 μmol/l	(3–17 μmol/l)
Alanine transaminase	23 IU/l	(5–35 IU/l)
Alkaline phosphatase	94 IU/l	(30–300 IU/l)
Gamma-glutamyl transpeptidase	36 IU/l	(11–51 IU/l)
Blood film	hypochromic, microcytic red cells	

A repeat endoscopy shows three duodenal ulcers in the first and second parts of the duodenum with histology showing no evidence of *Helicobacter pylori* infection.

QUESTIONS

- What is the likely diagnosis?
- How would you investigate and manage this patient?

ANSWER 90

This man presents with persistent upper abdominal pain. The pain of peptic ulceration is epigastric in position. In duodenal ulcer it usually precedes a meal and in gastric ulcer follows shortly after it. The pain is worsened by alcohol and spicy foods and eased by antacids and milk. The patient is tired because he has a microcytic anaemia due to slow upper gastrointestinal blood loss. The cause is presumed to be the persistent duodenal ulcer.

The differential diagnosis of recurrent peptic ulceration includes *Helicobacter pylori* ulcer disease, non-compliance or inadequate anti-ulcer treatment, a malignant ulcer and acute erosive ulceration often due to ingestion of non-steroidal anti-inflammatory drugs (NSAIDs). This man has peptic ulceration because of a **gastrin-secreting tumour**. The Zollinger–Ellison syndrome consists of severe peptic ulceration, hypersecretion of gastric acid and usually a gastrin-secreting islet cell tumour of the pancreas. The steady drive of hypergastrinaemia causes an increase in the parietal cell mass and consequent high basal and maximum acid secretion leading to aggressive peptic ulceration which may present with perforation or haemorrhage. The ulcers may occur in the distal duodenum or jejunum. Diarrhoea is characteristic because of the low intestinal pH denaturing pancreatic enzymes causing steatorrhoea and precipitating bile salts causing malabsorption in the colon.

Iron deficiency can be confirmed by measuring serum iron and total iron binding capacity or ferritin. In this patient fasting plasma gastrin levels were raised (> 50–100 pmol/l). Acid secretion should also be measured. Basal acid output is > 15 mmol/h, and is > 60 per cent of maximum acid output in this condition. The definitive test is a secretin test. After an intravenous injection of secretin the serum gastrin level normally falls, but in this patient it should rise > 50 per cent above normal levels. The tumour should be localized either by computed tomography (CT), arteriography or selective venous sampling. In this case a CT scan (Fig. 90.1) demonstrates a gastrinoma in the tail of the pancreas (arrow).

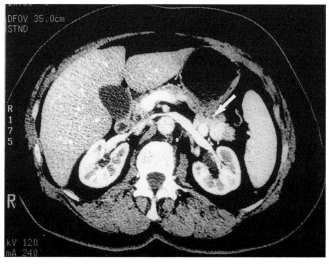

Figure 90.1 CT scan of pancreas

The patient should be given iron supplements and put on a maximum dose of a gastric proton-pump inhibitor to minimize gastric acid secretion. He should be referred to a specialist pancreatic surgeon. Although these tumours may metastasize to regional lymph nodes and the liver they are usually slow growing.

🔑 KEY POINTS

- If a patient has recurrent peptic ulceration non-compliance with treatment, *Helicobacter pylori* infection, NSAID use and Zollinger–Ellison syndrome should be considered.
- Ulcers in the distal duodenum and jejunum suggest excess gastrin secretion.

CASE 91

A 64-year-old woman is referred to outpatients with a six-month history of mild abdominal discomfort. This has been intermittent and involved the right iliac fossa mainly. There has been no particular relation to eating or to bowel movements. Over this time her appetite has gone down a little and she thinks that she has lost around 5 kg in weight. The intensity of the pain has become slightly worse over this time and it is now present on most days.

Over the last six weeks she has developed some new symptoms. She has developed a different sort of cramping abdominal pain located mainly in the right iliac fossa. This pain has been associated with a feeling of the need to pass her motions and often with some diarrhoea. During these episodes her husband has commented that she looked red in the face but she has associated this with the abdominal discomfort and the embarrassment from the urgent need to have her bowels open.

There is no other relevant previous medical history. She has smoked 15 cigarettes daily for the last 45 years and she drinks around 7 units of alcohol each week. She has noticed a little breathlessness on occasions over the last few months and has heard herself wheeze on several occasions. She has never had any problems with asthma and there is no family history of asthma or other atopic conditions.

She worked as a school secretary for 30 years and has never been involved in a job involving any industrial exposure. She has no pets. She has lived all her life in London and her only trip outside the UK was a day trip to France.

A computed tomography (CT) scan of her abdomen was performed and is shown in Fig. 91.1.

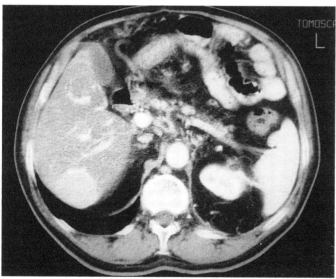

Figure 91.1 CT scan of abdomen

QUESTIONS

- What diagnoses should be considered?
- What investigations should be performed?

ANSWER 91

The symptoms she describes raise the possibility of a 5-hydroxytryptamine-secreting **carcinoid tumour**. The typical clinical features of the carcinoid syndrome are facial flushing, abdominal cramps and diarrhoea. Sometimes there is asthma and right-sided heart valve problems. The symptoms are characteristically intermittent and may come at times of increased release on activity. Skin changes may be persistent.

The CT scan of the liver shows a space-occupying lesion in the liver likely to represent a metastasis to the liver. Fluid-containing cystic lesions are of lower density. Other secondary tumours would give a similar appearance. Carcinoids do not generally produce their symptoms until they have metastasized to the liver from their original site which is usually in the small bowel. In the small bowel the tumours may produce local symptoms of obstruction or bleeding.

The symptoms of carcinoids are related to the secretion of 5-hydroxytryptamine (5-HT) by the tumour. The diagnosis depends on finding a high level of the metabolite 5-hydroxyindole acetic acid (5-HIAA) in a 24-hour collection of urine. Histology can be obtained from a liver biopsy guided to the correct area by ultrasound.

The symptoms can be controlled by antagonists of 5-HT such as cyproheptadine or by inhibitors of its synthesis p-chlorophenylalanine, or release, octreotide. The tumour can be reduced in size with consequent lessening of symptoms by embolization of its arterial supply using interventional radiology techniques.

When odd symptoms such as those described here occur the diagnosis of carcinoid tumour should always be remembered and investigated. In real life, most of the investigations for suspected carcinoid turn out to be negative.

Carcinoid tumours can occur in the lung when they act as slowly-growing malignant tumours. From the lung they can eventually be associated with left heart-valve problems. The other typical carcinoid features occur only after metastasis to the liver.

KEY POINTS

- Intermittent skin flushing, diarrhoea, wheezing and abdominal cramps are symptoms of the carcinoid syndrome.
- All these symptoms have much commoner causes.
- Metastasis to the liver (shown by ultrasound or CT) is present before the symptoms of carcinoid syndrome occur.

CASE 92

A 66-year-old man has been persuaded to go to his GP by his wife, having developed a change in character. His wife complains that over the last four weeks he has become lethargic and rather vague. He has a history of chronic cough and sputum production for the past 12 years. She thinks it was possible that these symptoms have increased a little over the previous eight weeks. He is a smoker of 20 cigarettes daily for 50 years, drinks around 14 units of alcohol per week and is on no medication. He had worked all his life as a postman until retirement six years ago.

On examination, he is a little vague in his answers to questions and has mild generalized muscle weakness. There are no abnormalities to find otherwise on physical examination. His peak flow and spirometry are within normal limits.

INVESTIGATIONS

		Normal
Haemoglobin	14.5 g/dl	13.0–17.0 g/dl
Mean corpuscular volume (MCV)	86 fl	80.5–99.7 fl
White cell count	6.5×10^9/l	$4.0–11.0 \times 10^9$/l
Platelet count	287×10^9/l	$150–400 \times 10^9$/l
Sodium	119 mmol/l	135–150 mmol/l
Potassium	3.4 mmol/l	3.4–5.0 mmol/l
Urea	3.2 mmol/l	2.5–7.5 mmol/l
Creatinine	64 μmol/l	70–120 μmol/l

His chest X-ray shown in Fig. 92.1.

QUESTIONS

- How do you interpret these findings?
- What would be the appropriate management?

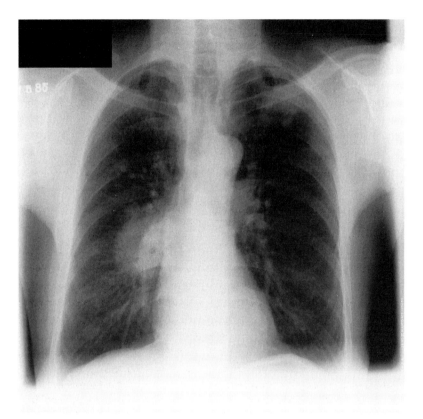

Figure 92.1 Chest X-ray

ANSWER 92

The blood results show hyponatraemia and the chest X-ray shows a mass overlying the right hilum. This degree of hyponatraemia might be expected to cause some cerebral changes. A lower level might be associated with fits. Above 120–125 mmol/l the effects are likely to be non-specific tiredness.

Possible causes for the hyponatraemia in this man are:

- **inappropriate antidiuretic hormone** (ADH) secretion found in association with the respiratory disorders of undifferentiated small cell carcinoma of the lung or, occasionally, with pneumonia or tuberculosis; and
- Addison's disease (adrenocortical failure) which would be expected to produce a high potassium level and postural hypotension. Addison's disease might be linked with respiratory problems through adrenal involvement by metastases or tuberculosis.

Other causes such as inappropriate ADH from drug therapy (e.g. carbamazepine, phenothiazines, amitriptyline), cerebrovascular events, salt-losing nephropathies or overhydration from intravenous fluids or overdrinking are not likely from the story given here. In view of the chest X-ray the most likely diagnosis is inappropriate ADH secretion with a small cell undifferentiated carcinoma of the lung. This can be confirmed by measurement of serum and urine osmolarities to show the serum dilution while the urine is concentrated. Levels of ADH (vasopressin) can be measured.

In this case, the osmolarities confirmed the syndrome of inappropriate ADH (SIADH) secretion; bronchial biopsies at fibreoptic bronchoscopy showed a small-cell undifferentiated carcinoma. Extension to the carina and CT appearances showed it to be not resectable. Fluid restriction to 750 ml daily produced an increase in serum sodium to 128 mmol/l with improvement in the confusion and weakness. If this fails to produce adequate results demeclocycline can be used. This derivative of tetracycline antibiotics interferes with the action of ADH in the renal tubules.

Chemotherapy was started for the lung tumour. Such treatment often produces a response in terms of shrinkage of the tumour, improved quality of life and increased survival. It may also help the ectopic hormone secretion. Unfortunately, cure is still infrequent. Small cell undifferentiated carcinomas of the lung are fast growing tumours, usually unresectable at presentation.

⚓ KEY POINTS

- Change of character may have a metabolic explanation.
- The commonest cause of hyponatraemia is diuretic therapy.
- Measurement of serum and urine osmolarities can help to determine the cause of hyponatraemia.

CASE 93

A 52-year-old man is brought to the casualty department by ambulance. His wife gives a history that, whilst standing at a bus stop, he fell to the ground and she was unable to rouse him. His breathing seemed to stop for about 20 s. He then developed jerking movements affecting his arms and legs lasting for about 2 min. She noticed that his face became blue and that he was incontinent of urine. He started to recover consciousness after a few minutes although he remains drowsy with a headache. The man has not complained of any symptoms prior to this episode. There is no significant past medical history. He is a taxi-driver. He smokes 20 cigarettes per day and consumes about three pints of beer each night.

On examination, he looks a fit and well-nourished man. He is afebrile. There is some bleeding from his tongue. His pulse is 84/min and regular. His blood pressure is 136/84. Examination of his heart, chest and abdomen is normal. There is no neck stiffness and there are no focal neurological signs. Fundoscopy is normal.

INVESTIGATIONS

		Normal
Haemoglobin	15.6 g/dl	(13.3–17.7g/dl)
Mean cell volume	85fl	(80–99fl)
White cell count	5.2×10^9/l	($3.9–10.6 \times 10^9$/l)
Platelets	243×10^9/l	($150–440 \times 10^9$/l)
Sodium	138 mmol/l	(135–145 mmol/l)
Potassium	4.8 mmol/l	(3.5–5.0 mmol/l)
Urea	6.2 mmol/l	(2.5–6.7 mmol/l)
Creatinine	76 μmol/l	(70–120 μmol/l)
Glucose	4.5 mmol/l	(4.0–6.0 mmol/l)
Calcium	2.25 mmol/l	(2.12–2.65 mmol/l)
Phosphate	1.2 mmol/l	(0.8–1.45 mmol/l)

QUESTIONS

- What are the differential diagnoses of this episode?
- How would you investigate and manage this man?
- What implications does the diagnosis have for this man's livelihood?

This man has had an episode characterized by sudden onset loss of consciousness associated with the development of generalized convulsions. The principal differential diagnosis is between an epileptic fit and a syncopal (fainting) attack. Syncope is a sudden loss of consciousness due to temporary failure of the cerebral circulation. Syncope is distinguished from a seizure principally by the circumstances in which the event occurs. For example, syncope usually occurs whilst standing, under situations of severe stress or in association with an arrhythmia. Sometimes a convulsion and urinary incontinence occur. Thus, neither of these is specific for an epileptic attack. The key is to establish the presence or absence of prodromal symptoms. Syncopal episodes are usually preceded by symptoms of dizziness and light-headedness. Other important neurological syndromes to exclude are transient ischaemic attacks, migraine, narcolepsy and hysterical convulsions. Transient ischaemic attacks are characterized by focal neurological signs and no loss of consciousness unless the vertebrobasilar territory is affected. The onset of migraine is gradual and consciousness is rarely lost. In narcolepsy consciousness is lost but convulsive movements are absent and the patient is easily wakened.

In this man's case the episode was witnessed by his wife who gave a clear history of a **grand mal (tonic–clonic seizure)**. There may be warning symptoms such as fear or an abnormal feeling referred to some part of the body – often the epigastrium – before consciousness is lost. The muscles become tonically contracted and the person will fall to the ground. The tongue may be bitten and there is usually urinary incontinence. Due to spasm of the respiratory muscles, breathing ceases and the subject becomes cyanosed. After this tonic phase, which can last up to a minute, the seizure passes into the clonic or convulsive phase. After the contractions end, the patient is stuporose which lightens through a stage of confusion to normal consciousness. There is usually a post-seizure headache and generalized muscular aches.

In adults, idiopathic epilepsy rarely begins after the age of 25 years. Blood tests should be performed to exclude metabolic causes such as hyponatraemia, hypoglycaemia and hypocalcaemia. Blood alcohol levels and gamma-glutamyltransferase levels should also be measured as markers of alcohol abuse. A computed tomography (CT) brain is needed to exclude a structural cause such as a brain tumour of cerebrovascular event. This man should be referred to a neurologist for further investigation including an EEG. This is necessary as he will probably not be able to continue in his occupation as a taxi-driver. Treatment with anticonvulsants for a single fit is also controversial.

⚒ Key Points

- It is vital to get an eye-witness account of a transient neurological episode to make a diagnosis.
- New onset epilepsy is rare in adults and should therefore be fully investigated to exclude an underlying cause.

CASE 94

A 23-year-old woman is admitted to the casualty department in a coma. The patient was found unconscious on the floor by her boyfriend. She had not been seen by anyone for the previous 48 hours. No history was available from the patient, but her partner volunteered the information that they were both intravenous heroin addicts. She is unemployed, smokes 25 cigarettes per day, drinks 40 units of alcohol per week and has used heroin for the past four years. They have occasionally shared needles with other addicts. They both had negative HIV tests about one year ago. She has not made any previous suicide attempts. She has had no other medical illnesses.

On examination, there are multiple old scarred needle puncture sites. Her pulse is 64/min regular, blood pressure 110/60, jugular venous pressure not raised, heart sounds normal. Her respiratory rate is 12/min, and she has dullness to percussion and bronchial breathing at the left base posteriorly. Abdominal examination is normal. Her conscious level is depressed but she is rousable to painful stimuli. She has pin-point pupils, but has no focal neurological signs. A bolus injection of intravenous naloxone causes her conscious level to rise transiently. Her left arm is swollen and painful from the shoulder down.

INVESTIGATIONS

		Normal
Haemoglobin	13.6 g/dl	(13.3–17.7g/dl)
White cell count	$9.2 \times 10^9/l$	$(3.9–10.6 \times 10^9/l)$
Platelets	$233 \times 10^9/l$	$(150–440 \times 10^9/l)$
Sodium	137 mmol/l	(135–145 mmol/l)
Potassium	7.8 mmol/l	(3.5–5.0 mmol/l)
Urea	42.3 mmol/l	(2.5–6.7 mmol/l)
Creatinine	622 μmol/l	(70–120 μmol/l)
Bicarbonate	14 mmol/l	(24–30 mmol/l)
Glucose	4.1 mmol/l	(4.0–6.0 mmol/l)
Calcium	1.64 mmol/l	(2.12–2.65 mmol/l)
Phosphate	3.6 mmol/l	(0.8–1.45 mmol/l)
Creatine kinase	68 000 i.u./l	(25–195 i.u./l)
Arterial blood gases (on air)		
pH	7.27	(7.38–7.44)
pco$_2$	7.5	(4.7–6.0 kPa)
po$_2$	9.2	(12.0–14.5 kPa)
Urinalysis	+protein;+++ blood.	
Urine microscopy	brown urine; no red cells; many granular casts	
ECG	flattened P wave; peaked T-waves	
Chest X-ray	extensive left lower-zone consolidation	

QUESTIONS

- What is the cause of this patient's acute renal failure?
- What further immediate and longer treatment does this woman need?

ANSWER 94

This patient has acute renal failure (high urea and creatinine levels) from **rhabdomyolysis**. Severe muscle damage causes a dramatically elevated creatine kinase, and a rise in serum potassium and phosphate levels. In this case, she has lain unconscious on her left arm for many hours due to an overdose of alcohol and intravenous heroin. As a result, she has developed severe ischaemic muscle damage causing release of myoglobin which is toxic to the kidneys. Other causes of rhabdomyolysis include crush injuries, severe hypokalaemia, excessive exercise, myopathies and certain viral infections. The urine is dark because of the presence of myoglobin which causes a false positive dipstick test for blood. Acute renal failure due to rhabdomyolysis causes profound hypocalcaemia in the oliguric phase due to calcium sequestration in muscle and reduced 1,25-dihydroxycalciferol levels, often with rebound hypercalcaemia in the recovery phase. This woman's conscious level is still depressed as a result of opiate and alcohol toxicity and she has clinical and radiological evidence of an aspiration pneumonia. She has a mixed metabolic and respiratory acidosis (low pH, bicarbonate) due to acute renal failure and respiratory depression ($p$co$_2$ elevated). Her arterial oxygenation is reduced due to hypoventilation and pneumonia. She also has a compartment syndrome in her arm due to massive swelling of her damaged muscles.

This patient has life-threatening hyperkalaemia with ECG changes. The ECG changes of hyperkalaemia progress from the earliest signs of peaking of the T-wave, P-wave flattening, prolongation of the PR interval through to widening of the QRS complex, a sine-wave pattern and ventricular fibrillation. Emergency treatment involves intravenous calcium gluconate which stabilizes cardiac conduction, and intravenous insulin/glucose, intravenous sodium bicarbonate and nebulized salbutamol, all of which temporarily lower the plasma potassium by increasing the cellular uptake of potassium. However, these steps should be regarded as holding measures whilst urgent dialysis is being organized.

The chest X-ray and clinical findings indicate consolidation of the left lower lobe. This patient should initially be managed on an intensive care unit. She will require antibiotics for her pneumonia and will require a naloxone infusion or mechanical ventilation for her respiratory failure. The patient should have vigorous rehydration with monitoring of her central venous pressure. If a good urinary flow can be maintained, urinary pH should be kept at < 7.0 by bicarbonate infusion which prevents the renal toxicity of myoglobin. This patient also needs to be considered urgently for surgical fasciotomy to relieve the compartment syndrome in her arm.

In the longer term, the patient needs counselling and with her boyfriend should be offered access to drug-rehabilitation services. They should also be offered testing for blood borne viruses (hepatitis B, C and HIV).

✎ KEY POINTS

- Acute hyperkalaemia is a life-threatening emergency.
- Aggressive fluid replacement and a forced alkaline diuresis can prevent renal damage in rhabdomyolysis if started early enough.

A 63-year-old man is admitted to hospital because of general fatigue, fever and weight loss. He has lost 10 kg in weight over the last six months. He has felt increasingly fatigued and has a very poor appetite. Over the past few weeks he has developed drenching night sweats. He has no chest pain or shortness of breath. His father died of pulmonary tuberculosis 30 years before. He has had no other serious medical illnesses. He is a widower and lives alone. He is a non-smoker and drinks no alcohol.

On examination, he is cachectic. His temperature is 38.0°C. There are no lymph nodes palpable. His conjunctivae are pale. Physical examination is otherwise normal.

INVESTIGATIONS

		Normal
Haemoglobin	7.6 g/dl	(13.3–17.7g/dl)
Mean cell volume	85 fl	(80–99 fl)
White cell count	12.2×10^9/l	($3.9–10.6 \times 10^9$/l)
Platelets	91×10^9/l	($150–440 \times 10^9$/l)
Erythrocyte sedimentation rate	120 mm/h	(<10 mm/h)
Sodium	136 mmol/l	(135–145 mmol/l)
Potassium	4.3 mmol/l	(3.5–5.0 mmol/l)
Urea	4.4 mmol/l	(2.5–6.7 mmol/l)
Creatinine	87 µmol/l	(70–120 µmol/l
Bilirubin	15 µmol/l	(3–17 µmol/l)
Alanine transaminase	26 IU/l	(5–35 IU/l)
Alkaline phosphatase	425 IU/l	(30–300 IU/l)

Blood film	immature red cells/nucleated red cells present
Serum electrophoresis	normal
Prostate-specific antigen	normal
Urinalysis	no protein; no blood
Chest X-ray	
Blood and urine cultures	negative

A chest X-ray is shown in Fig. 95.1.

QUESTIONS

- What is the diagnosis?
- How would you investigate and manage this patient?

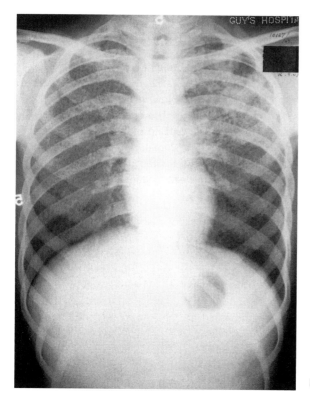

Figure 95.1 Chest X-ray

ANSWER 95

This patient has fever, marked weight loss, a leukoerythroblastic anaemia and a raised alkaline phosphatase. A very important finding is that immature red and white cells are seen in the peripheral blood. This leukoerythroblastic anaemia indicates bone-marrow replacement by tumour or infection forcing immature cells out into the blood. This man has **miliary tuberculosis**. Miliary tuberculosis is characterized by tuberculous granulomata throughout the body due to widespread dissemination of tubercle bacilli. It is now usually seen in elderly persons and the diagnosis is often only made at autopsy. The Chest X-ray may not always show miliary lesions (multiple small nodules about 2 mm in diameter). There may be choroidal tubercles in the eyes on fundoscopy and hepatosplenomegaly.

! DIFFERENTIAL DIAGNOSES OF FEVERS >3 WEEKS

- Other infections – visceral abscesses, infective endocarditis, specific organisms (e.g. brucellosis, actinomycosis or toxoplasmosis) and tropical diseases (e.g. malaria or trypanosomiasis).
- Neoplastic diseases – lymphomas, renal cell carcinomas, pancreatic tumours.
- Collagen vascular diseases, e.g systemic vasculitis, rheumatoid arthritis, systemic lupus erythematosus, temporal arteritis.
- Miscellaneous – recurrent pulmonary emboli, drug fever, sarcoidosis.

This patient needs an urgent diagnosis. Bronchoscopy with lavage may reveal acid-fast bacilli. Biopsy of his liver and bone marrow may show tubercle bacilli or caseating granulomas. The tissue should also be sent for culture. The tuberculin test may be negative because of immunoincompetence induced by the disease. Antituberculous treatment with three or four agents must be started immediately once biopsy material has been obtained. In severely ill patients corticosteroids are of benefit.

⚲ KEY POINTS

- Miliary tuberculosis is often missed as a cause of weight loss and fever in the elderly.
- Miliary tuberculosis may present with a leukoerythroblastic anaemia.
- Always culture biopsy material in patients with pyrexias of unknown origin.

A 38-year-old man presents to a neurologist having been referred because of memory loss and difficulty with concentration. He has recently lost his job as an accountant because of his increasingly poor performance at work. His wife and friends have noticed the decline in his memory for recent events over the past six months. The patient is sleeping poorly and has developed involuntary jerking movements of his limbs especially at night. He appears to his wife to be very short-tempered and careless of his personal appearance. He is married with two children and neither smokes tobacco nor drinks alcohol. He is not taking any regular medication. Aged 15, he received two years' treatment with growth hormone injections because of growth failure.

On physical examination, he is short but the examination is otherwise entirely normal other than the occasional myoclonic jerk affecting his legs. Fundoscopy is normal. Mental test scoring is grossly subnormal (3 out of 10).

MENTAL STATUS QUESTIONNAIRE

- What is the name of this place?
- What is the address of this place?
- What is the date?
- What month is it?
- What year is it?
- How old are you?
- When is your birthday?
- What year were you born?
- Who is the Prime Minister?
- Who was the previous Prime Minister?

QUESTIONS

- What is the diagnosis?
- What are the major differential diagnoses of this condition?
- How would you investigate and manage this patient?

ANSWER 96

The mental test score is very low at 3 out of 10, indicating severe impairment of cognitive function. A longer mini-mental state examination involves more questions scoring out of 30. The combination of a short history of rapidly advancing dementia often with focal neurological symptoms or signs would fit a diagnosis of **Creutzfeld–Jakob disease** (CJD). There may be focal or generalized fits and myoclonus is common. Speech may become severely affected and the patient may become mute. CJD may be familial or transmitted by prions by means of neurosurgical operations, corneal transplants or injections of growth hormone isolated from human pituitary glands. New variant CJD (nvCJD) is thought to be the human equivalent of bovine spongiform encephalopathy ('mad cow disease') due to ingestion of prions in infected cattle products. nvCJD often presents with psychiatric features and has characteristic neuropathological features.

Dementia is a progressive decline in mental ability affecting intellect, behaviour and personality. The earliest symptoms of dementia are an impairment of higher intellectual functions manifested by an inability to grasp a complex situation. Memory becomes impaired for recent events and there is usually increased emotional lability. In the later stages of dementia the patient becomes careless of appearance and eventually incontinent.

! CAUSES OF DEMENTIA

- Alzheimer's disease
- Multi-infarct dementia
- As part of progressive neurological diseases, e.g. multiple sclerosis.
- Normal pressure hydrocephalus – dementia, ataxia, urinary incontinence
- Neurosyphilis – general paralysis of the insane
- Vitamin B_{12} deficiency
- Intracranial tumours; subdural haematomas
- Hypothyroidism
- AIDS dementia

The investigations of this man should include a full blood count, erythrocyte sedimentation rate, serum urea and electrolytes, serum calcium, thyroid-function tests, liver-function tests, Venereal Disease Research Laboratory (VDRL) for syphilis, vitamin B_{12} and folic acid, HIV serology and computed tomography (CT) of the head. In CJD, the CT scan is usually normal, reflecting the rapid course of the disease with little time for atrophy.

There is no treatment for this condition. The neurologist must discuss with the family the diagnosis and prognosis. Counselling and support should be provided.

⚲ KEY POINTS

- Dementia at an early age requires rapid investigation to exclude a treatable cause.
- Most patients with presenile dementia have Alzheimer's disease.

CASE 97

A 48-year-old woman has complained of shortness of breath for three months. It has steadily become more severe and is associated with an occasional cough. Otherwise she has been well. She smokes 10 cigarettes per day and drinks about 10 units of alcohol each week. Her 20-year-old son has asthma and she has tried his salbutamol inhaler on two or three occasions but found it to be of no benefit. The shortness of breath tends to be worse on lying down but there are no other particular precipitating factors or variation through the day. She works as an office cleaner and has no significant previous medical history.

On examination, there is a generalized wheeze heard all over the chest but no other abnormal findings. She has tested herself on her son's peak flow meter at home and she has obtained values of about 100 l/min.

The chest X-ray is normal and she is sent for lung-function tests (Figs 97.1 and 97.2).

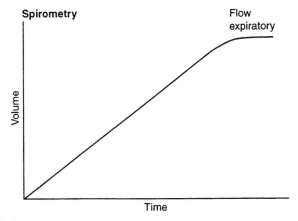

Figure 97.1 Spirometry

RESPIRATORY-FUNCTION TESTS

	Actual	Post bd	Predicted
FEV$_1$ (l)	1.20	1.20	3.5–4.3
FVC(l)	4.10	4.10	4.6–5.4
FER (FEV$_1$/FVC) (%)	29	29	72–80
PEF (l/min)	80	80	440–540
Residual volume (l)	1.8	1.8	1.6–2.8
Total lung capacity (l)	5.9	5.9	5.1–7.0

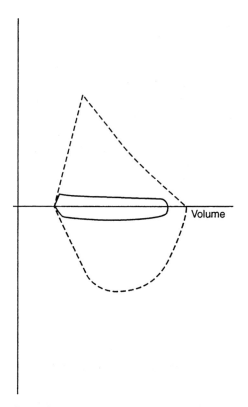

Figure 97.2 Flow–volume loop

- What do these findings indicate?

ANSWER 97

The flow–volume curve shows the same low flow throughout the whole volume of the vital capacity. It is similar in both inspiration and expiration as shown in the flow volume loop. This situation is typical of a rigid large airway obstruction. It is not reversible with bronchodilator therapy. The spirometry trace of volume against time in such cases shows a straight line of the same reduced flow right up to the vital capacity. These findings are typical of a narrowing in a larger airway (Figs 97.3 and 97.4). On examination, this airway narrowing is likely to produce a single monophonic wheeze which may be heard over a wide area of the chest.

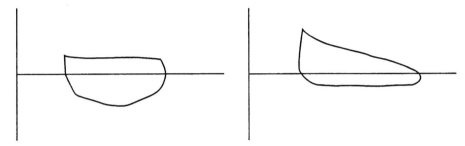

Figure 97.3 Intrathoracic narrowing   **Figure 97.4 Extrathoracic narrowing**

! DIFFERENTIAL DIAGNOSIS

The situation may easily be confused with asthma if the peak flow and the wheezing are accepted uncritically. In asthma, the spirometry will show a reduced FEV_1 but the flow rate (and therefore the slope of the line relating volume and time) will vary. The wheezing in asthma comes from many narrowed airways of different calibre and mass and the wheezes are often described as polyphonic.

The fixed flow in inspiration and expiration in this case suggest a rigid large airway narrowing. If the narrowing can vary a little with pressure changes, then the pattern will depend on the site of the narrowing. If it is outside the thoracic cage, as in a laryngeal lesion, it will be more evident on inspiration. If the site is intrathoracic, the flow limitation will be greater in expiration. Large airway narrowing can be caused by inflammatory conditions such as tuberculosis or Wegener's granulomatosis, damage from prolonged endotracheal intubation or by extrinsic pressure such as a retrosternal goitre. However, the commonest cause is a **carcinoma of a large airway**.

Some further investigation of the large airways is required. In the presence of a normal chest X-ray this could be a bronchoscopy or a computed tomography (CT) scan. A bronchoscopy to see and biopsy any lesion would be best. In this case, fibreoptic bronchoscopy showed a carcinoma in the lower trachea reducing the lumen to a small orifice. Treatment was by radiotherapy with oral steroids to cover any initial swelling of the tumour which might increase the degree of obstruction in the trachea

A 22-year-old woman is referred to a dermatologist complaining of increasing growth of hair affecting her face. This has progressed over at least two years so that now she needs to shave to remove her facial hair. She has also noticed facial acne and that her skin is more greasy. Her periods have become very irregular with her last period being three months previously. Her menarche was at age 13, but over the past three years her periods have been very erratic with her intermenstrual interval ranging from a few days to many months and her blood loss varying from light to heavy. She has had no significant medical illnesses previously. She lives alone, smokes 20 cigarettes per week and drinks about 20 units of alcohol per week. She is taking no regular medication.

On examination she is overweight at 16 stone. Her facial skin is greasy and she has excessive facial hair. Physical examination is otherwise normal.

ENDOCRINE INVESTIGATIONS

		Normal
Follicle-stimulating hormone (FSH)	1 U/l	(2–8U/l)
Luteinizing hormone (LH)	32 U/l	(6–13U/l)
Oestradiol	284 nmol/24h	(10–55 nmol/l)
Testosterone	9.6 nmol/l	(1–2.1 nmol/l)

QUESTIONS

- What is the diagnosis?
- How would you investigate and manage this patient?

ANSWER 98

This patient has hirsutism and secondary amenorrhoea due to **polycystic ovaries** (Stein–Leventhal syndrome). This is a complex disorder characterized by excessive androgen production by the ovaries and/or adrenal cortex which interferes with ovarian follicular ripening. A large number of follicles develop abnormally leading to enlarged ovaries. Patients are usually obese with the adipose tissue converting androgens to oestrogens leading to high LH levels stimulated by positive feedback of oestrogens on the pituitary, and low FSH levels due to negative feedback. The low FSH level means that ovarian follicles do not mature normally. Reduction of sex hormone-binding globulin is induced by testosterone increasing the active fraction of circulating testosterone.

! DIFFERENTIAL DIAGNOSES OF HIRSUTISM

- Constitutional
- Drugs, e.g. cyclosporin, minoxidil
- Cushing's syndrome
- Congenital adrenal hyperplasia
- Androgen-secreting tumours
- Hypothyroidism

Patients with androgenic tumours usually have a shorter history, signs of virilism such as clitoral hypertrophy and very high testosterone levels.

This woman had an ovarian ultrasound (Fig. 98.1) which showed polycystic ovaries (a cyst indicated by an arrow). A laparoscopic biopsy confirmed the diagnosis. Hirsutism can be treated by combined oestrogen/progestogen oral contraception (to induce sex hormone-binding globulin and thus mop up excess unbound testosterone) and by the anti-androgen, cyproterone acetate. Ovulation can be induced with clomiphene or pulsatile Gondotrophin-releasing hormone (GnRH) therapy. Dietary advice should be given to reduce obesity which otherwise helps maintain the condition.

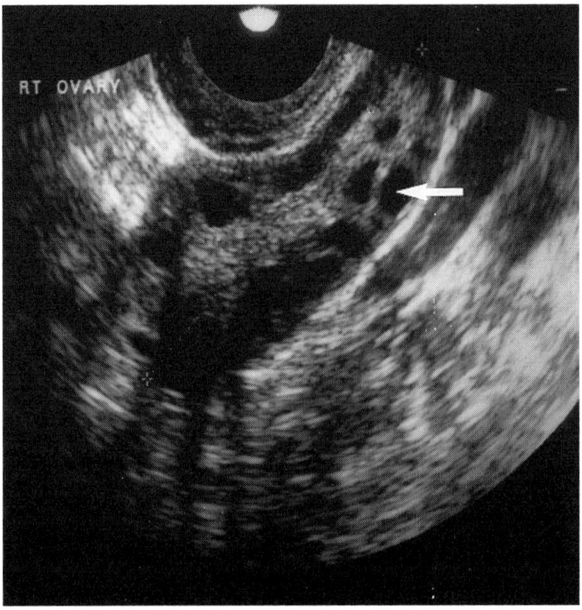

Figure 98.1 Ovarian ultrasound

- True hirsutism is due to excessive androgens, whereas constitutional hirsutism is found in certain ethnic groups.
- Associated menstrual irregularities and obesity is suggestive of true hirsutism and polycystic ovary syndrome.

A 35-year-old woman has a year long history of intermittent diarrhoea which has never been bad enough for her to seek medical help in the past. However, she has become much worse over one week with episodes of bloody diarrhoea ten times a day. She has had some crampy lower abdominal pain which lasts for 1–2 hours and is partially relieved by defaecation. Over the last 2–3 days she has become weak with the persistent diarrhoea and her abdomen has become more painful and bloated over the last 24 hours.

She has no relevant previous medical history. Up to one year ago, her bowels were regular. There is no disturbance of micturition or menstruation. In her family history, she thinks one of her maternal aunts may have had bowel problems. She has two children aged 3 and 8 years. They are both well. She travelled to Spain on holiday six months ago but has not travelled elsewhere.

She smokes 10 cigarettes a day and drinks rarely. She took 2 days of amoxycillin after the diarrhoea began with no improvement or worsening of her bowels.

On examination her blood pressure is 108/66. Her pulse rate is 110/min, respiratory rate 18/min. Her abdomen is rather distended and tender generally, particularly in the left iliac fossa. Faint bowel sounds are audible.

The abdominal X-ray shows a dilated colon with no faeces.

BLOOD TESTS

		Normal
Haemoglobin	11.1 g/dl	11.7–15.7 g/dl
Mean corpuscular volume (MCV)	79 fl	80.8–100 fl
White cell count	8.8×10^9/l	$3.5–11.0 \times 10^9$/l
Platelet count	280×10^9/l	$150–440 \times 10^9$/l
Sodium	139 mmol/l	135–145 mmol/l
Potassium	3.3 mmol/l	3.5–5.0 mmol/l
Urea	7.6 mmol/l	2.5–6.7 mmol/l
Creatinine	89 μmol/l	70–120 μmol/l

QUESTIONS

- What is your interpretation of these results?
- What is the likely diagnosis and what should be the management?

ANSWER 99

Bloody diarrhoea ten times a day suggests a serious active colitis. In the absence of any recent foreign travel it is most likely that this is an acute episode of **ulcerative colitis** on top of chronic involvement. The dilated colon suggests a diagnosis of toxic megacolon which can rupture with potentially fatal consequences. Investigations such as sigmoidoscopy and colonoscopy may be dangerous in this acute situation and should be deferred until there has been reasonable improvement. The blood results show a microcytic anaemia suggesting chronic blood loss and low potassium from diarrhoea and raised urea from fluid loss.

If the history was just the acute symptoms, then infective causes of diarrhoea would be higher in the differential diagnosis. Nevertheless, stool should be examined for ova, parasites and culture. Inflammatory bowel disorders have a familial incidence but the woman has an unknown condition and the relationship is not close enough to be helpful in diagnosis. Smoking is associated with Crohn's disease but ulcerative colitis is more common in non-smokers.

She should be treated immediately with corticosteroids and intravenous fluid replacement. If the colon is increasing in size or is initially larger than 5.5 cm then a laparotomy should be performed to remove the colon. If not, the steroids should be continued until the symptoms resolve and diagnostic procedures such as colonoscopy and biopsy can be carried out safely. Sulphasalazine or mesalazine are used in the chronic maintenance treatment of ulcerative colitis after resolution of the acute attack.

In this case, the colon steadily enlarged despite fluid replacement and other appropriate treatment. She required surgery with a total colectomy and ileo-rectal anastomosis. The histology confirmed ulcerative colitis. The ileorectal anastomosis will be reviewed regularly.

KEY POINTS

- Bloody diarrhoea implies serious colonic pathology.
- It is important to monitor colonic dilatation carefully in colitis and vital to operate before rupture.
- Both Crohn's disease and ulcerative colitis can cause a similar picture of active colitis.

An 18-year-old woman is admitted to accident & emergency complaining of severe vertigo. This has developed over the past few hours and previously she was well. She has the sensation of her surroundings spinning around her. She feels nauseated and sleepy. She does not have a headache. The patient has not had any previous medical illnesses. She is a non-smoker, does not drink alcohol and is taking no regular medication. She lives with her parents and is due to sit her A-levels in three weeks. Her father suffers from epilepsy and her mother has hypothyroidism.

On examination, she is drowsy and her speech is slurred. Her pulse rate is 64/min, blood pressure 90/70 and respiratory rate 12/min. Examination of her cardiovascular, respiratory and abdominal systems is otherwise normal. Her peripheral nervous system examination is normal apart from impaired coordination and a staggering gait. Fundoscopy is normal. Her pupils are equal and reacting. There is a normal range of eye movements but she has multidirectional nystagmus. Her hearing is normal as is the rest of her cranial nerve examination.

QUESTIONS

- What is the diagnosis?
- What are the major differential diagnoses of vertigo?
- How would you manage this patient?

ANSWER 100

The acute onset of these symptoms and signs with drowsiness in an 18-year-old girl raise the possibility of a drug overdose. Her father is epileptic and is likely to be taking anticonvulsants. This patient has taken a **phenobarbitone overdose**, tablets which her father uses to control his epilepsy. She has taken an overdose as a result of concern about her imminent exams. Excessive ingestion of barbiturates, alcohol and phenytoin all cause acute neurotoxicity manifested by vertigo, dysarthria, ataxia and nystagmus. In severe cases coma, respiratory depression and hypotension occur.

Vertigo is an awareness of disordered orientation of the body in space and takes the form of a sensation of rotation of the body or its surroundings.

! CAUSES OF VERTIGO

Peripheral lesions	Central lesions
Benign positional vertigo	Brainstem ischaemia
Vestibular neuronitis	Posterior fossa tumours
Ménière's disease	Multiple sclerosis
Middle-ear diseases	Alcohol/drugs
Aminoglycoside toxicity	Migraine; epilepsy

The duration of attacks is helpful in distinguishing some of these causes of vertigo. Benign positional vertigo lasts less than one minute. Attacks of Ménière's disease are recurrent and last up to 24 hours. Vestibular neuronitis does not recur but lasts several days, whereas vertigo due to ototoxic drugs is usually permanent. Brainstem ischaemic attacks occur in patients with evidence of diffuse vascular disease and long tract signs may be present. Multiple sclerosis may initially present with an acute attack of vertigo that lasts for two to three weeks. Posterior fossa tumours usually have symptoms and signs of space-occupying lesions. Acoustic neuromas often present with vertigo and deafness. Migrainous attacks are often accompanied by nausea and vomiting. Temporal lobe epilepsy may also produce rotational vertigo, often associated with auditory and visual hallucinations. Central lesions produce nystagmus which is multidirectional and may be vertical. Peripheral lesions induce a unilateral horizontal nystagmus.

The diagnosis in this case can be made by measuring plasma phenobarbitone levels and by asking the patient's father to check if his tablets are missing. Gastric lavage should be carried out if it is within 12 hours of ingestion of the tablets. A forced alkaline diuresis is indicated for serious barbiturate overdoses and charcoal haemoperfusion (if available) can also be used. National Poisons Information Services are available to advise on treatment. Before discharge she should have counselling and treatment by adolescent psychiatrists.

🔍 KEY POINTS

- Vertigo can be caused by a variety of neurological disorders.
- A careful history and examination may reveal the cause of vertigo.

INDEX

Italic type refers to symptoms and **bold type** indicates diagnosed conditions. Capitals refer to major body systems.

269

epilepsy 248
erythema nodosum 32

facial acne 261
facial hair 261
fainting 217
falls 147
familial hypercholesterolaemia 236
fatigue 1, 249
fever 41, 43, 127, 251
food poisoning 20
fracture 109

gastrin-secreting tumour 238
GASTROENTEROLOGY, see cases on pages
  19, 39, 73, 107, 129, 151, 157, 173, 189,
  209, 219, 229, 241, 265
grand mal (tonic-clonic seizure) 248

haematemesis 107
haematuria 51, 211
HAEMATOLOGY, see cases on pages 67, 109,
  153, 187, 213, 231, 251
haemochromatosis 176
Haemophilus influenzae 30, 143, 144
haemorrhoids 220
hand enlargement 59
headache 29, 55, 59, 69, 75, 85, 129, 187,
  191, 231
Helicobacter pylori 74, 237, 238
hepatolenticular degeneration 222
hirsutism 262
HIV seroconversion illness 44
hypercalcaemia 110, 116, 197, 204
hyperglycaemic ketoacidotic coma 170
hypertension 23, 55, 113, 179, 215
hyperthyroidism 126
hypertrophic pulmonary osteoarthropathy
  (HPOA) 48
hypothermia 136, 137
hypothyroidism 2, 37, 156, 220

IgA nephropathy 212
inappropriate antidiuretic hormone (ADH)
  244
INFECTIOUS DISEASES, see cases on pages
  43, 127, 139
infective endocarditis 202
intra-abdominal sepsis 226
irritability 125
irritable bowel syndrome (IBS) 69, 130

ischaemic bowel 210
ischaemic heart disease 72
itching 113, 187

jaundice 155, 221, 225
joint pain 63, 123, 175, 183, 195

leg weakness 141
lethargy 243
leukaemia 154
libido loss 175
LIVER, see cases on pages 77, 79, 155, 175,
  221
loin pain 51
loss of appetite 55
loss of consciousness 7, 21
lymphoma 154

macrocytic anaemia 232
malaise 79, 201, 221
malaria 128
malignant melanoma 82
Mallory–Weiss lesion 108
memory loss 255
metabolic acidosis 162
METABOLIC DISORDERS, see cases on
  pages 23, 55, 83, 115, 161, 169, 203,
  235
microcytic anaemia 74
microscopic haematuria 211
miliary tuberculosis 253
mitral stenosis 34
monoarthritis 16
monoarthropathy 16
motor neuropathy 142
multiple myeloma 110
muscle cramps 55
muscle pain 123
muscle stiffness 103, 215
muscle weakness 161, 163, 243
myasthenia gravis 164
mycobacterium avium complex (MAC) 140
Mycobacterium tuberculosis 76, 190

nausea 77, 113, 115
Neisseria meningitidis 30
nephrotic syndrome 12
neurogenic diabetes insipidus 204
NEUROLOGY, see cases on pages 29, 69, 95,
  141, 163, 215, 247, 255, 267
night sweats 85